THE BODYWORK AND MASSAGE SOURCEBOOK

THE BODYWORK AND MASSAGE SOURCEBOOK

ANDREW S. LEVINE, L.M.T.
VALERIE J. LEVINE, PH.D.

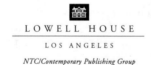

LOWELL HOUSE

LOS ANGELES

NTC/Contemporary Publishing Group

Library of Congress Cataloging-in-Publication Data

Levine, Andrew S.
    The bodywork and massage sourcebook / Andrew S. Levine, Valerie J. Levine.
        p.   cm.
    Includes bibliographical references and index.
    ISBN 0-7373-0098-1
    1. Massage.   2. Mind and body therapies.   I. Levine, Valerie J.   II. Title.
RA780.5.L48   1999
615.8'22—dc21   99-14297
                                                                                          CIP

Text Design by Laurie Young

Published by Lowell House
A division of NTC/Contemporary Publishing Group, Inc.
4255 West Touhy Avenue, Lincolnwood (Chicago), Illinois 60646-1975 U.S.A.

Printed in the United States of America
International Standard Book Number: 0-7373-0098-1
99 00 01 02 03 04 RRD 18 17 16 15 14 13 12 11 10 9 8 7 6 5 4 3 2 1

To our parents,

Shirley and Herbert Levine and Rochelle and Simpson Sasserath,

for their unconditional love and support.

Acknowledgments

We would like to thank our colleagues, other professionals, and friends for their support and contributions to this book.

The editors, Bud Sperry, Maria Magallanes, and Jama Carter

Brian and Mary Hade, Core Therapeutics

Adrienne Rodewald

Robert Blasi

Carol Klebacher

Edward Feldman, D.C.

Betty Post

Caroline May

Sue Brenner, Rosen Center East

Kim Buckalew

Cheryl Mulligan

Andrew Levine's teachers at the Somerset School of Massage Therapy:

> Bob and Susen Edwards
>
> Toni Smith
>
> Stella Rojas
>
> Brian Smith
>
> Ron Diana
>
> Jan Saunders
>
> Guy DeRosa

Contents

Introduction

Human touch has the power to heal. Bodywork and massage provide theoretical frameworks, guiding principles, and specific techniques that harness the power of touch to enhance your physical and mental health. The purpose of this book is to provide you with information on a variety of massage and bodywork modalities so that you can make informed choices.

This book is coauthored by a licensed massage therapist (Andrew Levine) and a licensed psychologist (Valerie Levine) who are also husband and wife. We would like to begin by sharing with you the evolution of our interest in massage and bodywork.

ABOUT THE AUTHORS

Andy's Story

When I was about seven years old, my mom used to say to me, "Son, please rub your mother's aching feet." As I massaged her feet she would say, "That feels so good, Andrew. You have wonderful hands. Maybe you will become a podiatrist when you grow up." Although I had no idea what a podiatrist was, I knew my mother was paying me a compliment. I also had no idea that after taking a circuitous route, I would eventually become a professional massage therapist.

As a teenager and young adult, I was involved in athletics, and I placed a great deal of value on the optimal functioning of my muscles. But as a college student living away from home, I was not yet focused on how I could channel my interests and talents into a satisfying profession.

After college, I played it safe and went directly into the family business. It never really occurred to me to do anything else. My dad owned a large industrial laundry with route service and lots of employees. As the customer service representative, I worked long hours and took on the least desirable tasks.

At age twenty-seven I bought a dry-cleaning plant and was ready to shine as an entrepreneur. I built a large business with four stores and about twenty-five employees. I was good with my hands and took care of the garments that needed special treatments. Unfortunately, the corrosive chemicals were harming my hands, not to mention my lungs. There were other problems. The government was overregulating the industry. Tired, frustrated customers would complain bitterly over a missed stain or misplaced order. Yet, when the work was perfect, compliments were few. My satisfaction with work diminished. I allowed myself to face what I always knew somewhere in my mind—that following in my father's footsteps was not what I really wanted to do.

I decided to sell the business before I turned forty. At age thirty-nine, I was no longer owned by my business. I was free. But I was also jobless.

After all of this, I was still looking for managerial and sales positions. Hadn't I learned anything about following my own heart?

My wife (and coauthor), Valerie, a psychologist, would come home after a long day with pain in her upper back and cramps in her feet. Like my mother, Valerie would remark about my intuitive touch. She suggested that it was time I combine my natural talents and nurturing temperament with formal training and consider massage therapy as a profession.

I had been out of school for seventeen years and was nervous about pursuing a career so different from what I had done before. But a lightbulb went off in my head—I could apply everything I had done before and finally do something I love. I could use my hands to heal. The desire to take the risk became powerful. I made an appointment for an interview at the Somerset School of Massage Therapy, the most respected and fully accredited massage therapy school in New Jersey.

As I underwent the application and interview process and took a tour of the school, I felt increasingly confident that I had made the right choice. I paid my first tuition and bought all my books on the spot, eagerly awaiting the orientation.

School was challenging and fast-paced. My classmates and I worked well together. There was a wealth of diverse information to absorb and apply. I discovered that massage is a complex area involving the body, the mind, physical and mental health, and a way of looking at life. I was able to combine the technical knowledge with my natural intuition. I discovered and studied many massage and bodywork modalities. The more I learned, the more I changed, becoming the person I deep down always wanted to be.

My personal triumph came at the end of the program. The treatment of a fellow student was our final hands-on exam. One of my classmates had coincidentally thrown his back out while assembling something at home. He was in such pain that he had been unable to give or even receive massage for over a week. Calling on my newly acquired assessment and treatment skills, I configured a treatment plan and used all the tools in my repertoire to help my comrade. He rose from the table one hour later *pain-free.* Both of us were astounded.

Since that time, I have built a successful practice as a massage therapist. I have learned that, even though I cannot help everyone, I have provided pain relief and changed lives. I treat each client as an individual and perform an assessment before deciding on an approach.

Massage school was just the beginning. Learning more about massage and bodywork is an ongoing part of my life. My excitement about my work and my desire to communicate about the significance and diversity of massage and bodywork led me to write this book.

Valerie's Story

I can still picture myself sitting at the immobile wooden desk in elementary school and reaching around my neck to rub my upper back between my shoulder blades. My massage therapist (before my husband), Adrienne Rodewald, acknowledged and helped relieve my pain about thirty years after I began to experience it. She called the affected region my "responsibility area." I immediately understood what she meant. I burdened myself with so much responsibility that the weight of it on my shoulders and back was hurting me physically. She lovingly explained to me that almost all the therapists she massaged held their stress and feelings in hidden areas, especially the neck and upper back.

I discovered massage and bodywork just a few years after being in private practice as a psychologist. All the muscular discomfort I experienced up until that time became compounded by doing a lot of sitting and listening. For more than the past ten years, I have received massage and bodywork, at first for relief from muscle tension and later for such additional benefits as a closer integration of body and mind and the maintaining of homeostasis, a balanced state. I have also had personal insights and made good decisions during the process of massage.

Adrienne recently told me, "You would be upset about something. You would verbalize about it during the massage—which is not everyone's experience. And you would have the answer by the end of the massage. And sometimes it was not at all what you thought it was going to be. I was just listening as you were figuring it out. And that was pretty amazing, knowing your field."

Having massage and bodywork in my life has made me more spontaneous, productive, and happy. It has made me a more relaxed and open person and a more holistically oriented therapist. I have often recommended various forms of massage and bodywork to my clients as an adjunct to psychotherapy.

My interest in coauthoring this book stems from my enjoyment of massage and bodywork, as well as a deep interest in mind-body interaction and the impact of the mind-body system on mental and physical health. I believe that no matter how much psychotherapy an individual undertakes, long-term recovery and growth cannot be fully achieved if the body is ignored, neglected, or unappreciated. Psychotherapy and massage therapy make for a natural marriage.

ABOUT THIS BOOK

In this first section of the book, we will make you aware of how the power of touch provided by bodywork and massage can improve the quality of your life. Once you understand how touch enhances the body and the mind, you will be ready to begin your exploration of the exciting modalities chosen for this book. The chapters in this first section include:

- The Power of Touch
- Bodywork/Massage and Your Health
- The Giver/Receiver Relationship
- Bodywork and Massage Modalities

At the end of the book, you will find a two-part appendix with useful information. The contents of the appendices are as follows:

Appendix A provides a summary in easy-to-read form of the key features of the bodywork/massage modalities described in the book. Examining the key features will help you compare the modalities on many dimensions, from depth of touch to amount of clothing worn to length of session. As you might expect, cost will vary to some extent depending on your geographical location and the practitioner you choose.

Appendix B is a resource for obtaining more information about the modalities covered in this book. The organizations listed can help you locate qualified bodywork practitioners and massage therapists who practice the various modalities in your geographical area. Addresses and phone numbers of key associations and institutions are provided. It is important to select a bodywork practitioner or massage therapist with as much care as you have selected other professionals who have provided you with individually tailored services that impact your life and well-being.

If you would like to do further reading on massage and bodywork in general or on a particular modality, you might find books and articles of interest in the bibliography included at the end of the book.

CHAPTER 1

The Power of Touch

Bodywork, which includes massage therapy, is a form of communication through touch. Although the nature of hands-on touch may differ from one modality to another, all types of bodywork and massage have the perspective that human touch communicates positive, soothing messages to both the body and the mind.

Touch messages are real. They are transmitted to the brain via nerve endings where chemicals are released that signal the muscles to relax. This physical release is accompanied by feelings of well-being and more optimal overall functioning.

Touch is the first sense to develop in human beings. Human, nurturing touch is so essential that babies will fail to thrive and eventually die without it, even if they are provided with proper nutrition. Although as adults, we will not die without nurturing touch, we thrive with it. Massage and bodywork can provide the kinds of touch that help *prevent* physical and emotional problems and help *heal* the body and the mind.

TOUCH AFFECTS US ON MANY LEVELS

The touch in bodywork and massage, whether light or deep, can promote healing on a number of levels. The depth of touch is not necessarily an accurate gauge as to depth of impact. Modalities based on light, gentle strokes and movements can have a profound effect on physical and mental health.

On the physical level, the healing power of touch may result in your feeling less pain in your shoulder, resulting in freer movement, or the release of long-standing tightness in your chest, resulting in freer breathing. On the mental and emotional levels, touch heals by facilitating mental clarity, improving concentration, alleviating stress, reducing anxiety, and fighting depression. The touch provided in massage and bodywork can help you feel more comfortable with yourself and with your body, factors that contribute to healthy self-esteem.

Appropriate touch also enhances positive communication between the body and the mind. The relationship between internal bodily and mental processes is at the heart of the mechanism through which touch derives its power.

THE MIND-BODY FEEDBACK LOOP

The internal reaction triggered by touch affects communication throughout the mind-body feedback loop. Here is how the loop works:

Mental tension created by circular obsessive thought patterns, also known as worrying, makes your muscles tense. Your tense muscles signal your brain, creating further mental tension. Your whole being becomes uptight.

You decide to get a massage.

The process of therapeutic, nurturing touch can break this pattern by providing touch signals that communicate "Relax" to the mind, as well as to the body. Once relaxed, the mind and body can communicate with each other more openly and efficiently by providing equally powerful messages to relax and move freely.

Touch has the power to help you substitute a positive mind-body feedback loop for the negative one that was maintaining your stress. The refreshing, open flow of communication within the mind-body system promotes creativity, spontaneity, and a feeling of relaxed vitality.

THE POWER OF TOUCH THROUGHOUT HISTORY

The significance and healing power of human touch has been acknowledged for thousands of years. Massage, the systematic rubbing and manipulation of the tissues of the body, is one of the oldest means used for the relief of bodily infirmities. Massage has been in recorded existence since the year 2200 B.C. Eastern cultures are way ahead of Western cultures in the realization that human touch is a powerful tool for improving physical health and promoting feelings of well-being. There would be no modern forms of massage and bodywork without the foundation laid by Eastern cultures.

As long ago as about 1800 B.C., the Ayurveda, the earliest known medical text from India, listed massage as a primary healing practice. Massage has been practiced in India and Japan for many centuries. Massage was practiced by the Greeks and Romans in connection with their therapeutic baths. Herodotus taught Hippocrates massage and medical gymnastics. Julius Caesar, who suffered from epilepsy, had himself pinched all over and massaged on a daily basis. Through the power of touch, he was better able to carry on his work.

A percussive type of touch, known as whipping, was used by the ancient Roman physicians to treat a variety of diseases and is still used by Laplanders and Finns who beat the body with bundles of birch twigs. The natives of the South Pacific islands have used massage for hundreds of years.

The Chinese practiced massage as many as three thousand years ago. In fact, an ancient Chinese book that was later translated into French was probably the foundation for the Swedish massage strokes developed and systematized by Per Henrik Ling in the 1830s, which in turn became the basis of modern massage. In France and other European countries, massage has been a popular treatment for pulled muscles since the nineteenth century.

THE PERCEPTION OF TOUCH IN AMERICA TODAY

Mixed feelings and mixed messages about touch between human beings are prevalent in America today. Not everyone perceives human physical contact in the same way. Individuals vary in their use of casual touch in social situations. Many Americans shy away from touch.

Clearing up Misconceptions

In the case of massage, there still exists a misconception in our culture that the underlying intent of the process is sexual rather than therapeutic. The reality is that sexual touch is in no way a part of therapeutic touch. The significance of appropriate boundaries in the relationship between the giver and receiver of touch and how to create and maintain such boundaries are topics covered in the training of massage therapists and bodywork practitioners.

Establishing appropriate boundaries and knowledge of personal rights are essential in the giving and receiving of massage and bodywork. It is important that you, as the client, understand that you can say no to being touched by anyone at any time, and your wishes should be respected. Worrying about offending the practitioner should not prevent you from expressing discomfort or changing your mind. Americans' ambivalence about the acceptability of touch is probably why it has taken so long to integrate legitimate, nurturing touch practices into our lives.

Touch Deprivation

Hand in hand with the confusion and taboos, there is a compelling desire on the part of most people to be touched in a way that makes them feel good. In fact, adults crave touch. In its absence, some individuals choose poor substitutes, like too much food or alcohol. What they really want is nurturing touch.

Research has shown that friends and family members in European countries touch each other significantly more frequently during social interaction than do American friends and families. The taboo against touching in the course of everyday life may be causing touch deprivation.

America is what anthropologists call a "nontactile" society as compared with most other cultures. In "The Magic of Touch: Massage's Healing Powers Make It Serious Medicine," an article in the Discovery section of *Life* magazine (August 1997), Tiffany Field, Ph.D., expresses concern that Americans are not getting enough touch, especially with increased attention on sexual harassment and abuse in schools and in the workplace. Touch is even taboo in preschools between teacher and child. Field observes, "America is suffering from an epidemic of skin hunger." She believes that touch has a strong impact on the growth, development, and well-being of children and that touch is an essential part of daily life for all of us.

The absence of touch contributes to the emptiness and lack of connection with the world that so many people experience in today's high-paced, technological society. Being starved for consistent, nurturing touch may even account, to some extent, for the pervasiveness of anxiety, stress, depression, aggression, and even heart disease, which are so much a part of American culture today.

TOUCH MESSAGES FOR CHILDREN

Touch is not a simple issue for children in today's society. Given the horrendous acts committed against children and the lengths to which we must go to protect them, many children are confused about touch.

Good Touch and Bad Touch

On the one hand, we encourage our children to be kind, caring, and loving individuals. We want them to feel free to express and be themselves. On the other hand, we are forced to teach them, even rehearse them, to be wary of strangers, even those strangers who appear on the surface to be nice people.

We are afraid, and make them afraid, that they might be touched in a way that is harmful, even deadly. We are forced to communicate this message to children as early as preschool, the first point in their lives when they are out of their parents' sight.

Preschool children are taught about *good touch* and *bad touch*. As children get older, the education about good and bad touch becomes more detailed, and no less confusing. It is difficult for most children to sort out how to be a friendly, helpful, loving person but run from a stranger who looks like a nice person or even asks for the child's help.

Some children grow up in environments in which nurturing touch is a part of everyday life. Others are deprived of touch and physical affection. Unfortunately, there are some who are exposed to traumatic touch from physical or sexual abuse. If a child has already experienced bad touch, teaching appropriate touch and boundary messages is even more challenging for parents.

Providing Healthy Messages

Touch issues affect all of us throughout our lifetime. Children who learn healthy views of touch and are provided with positive tactile experiences by their caregivers are the most likely to grow up to be adults with good self-esteem, a sense of appropriate boundaries, and long-lasting intimate relationships.

What can parents do to provide healthy messages about touch and to encourage children to welcome nurturing, appropriate touch into their lives?

1. By more than any other means, children learn and internalize what they see and how they are treated in their environments on a consistent basis. Parents can provide healthy touch messages by being good role models for touch by showing spontaneous physical affection in the form of casual touching and hugging with each other, with their children, and among family members and friends.

2. It is important that parents educate their children with sensitivity about how to keep themselves safe from unwelcome and potentially dangerous touch.

3. Parents should remember to respect their children's privacy and requests not to be touched, tickled, or physically handled in any way that is uncomfortable for that individual child.

4. Probably the best way to instill in your children safe, positive messages about touch is to massage them on a regular basis, starting when they are babies. Stimulating your child's developing nervous system in this way and providing the pleasurable trusting feelings that accompany infant massage will provide you and your child with a good foundation for dealing with a whole array of touch issues throughout your child's journey into adulthood. Infant massage is covered in chapter 6 of this book.

THE CURRENT STATUS OF MASSAGE

It is only in recent generations that the practices of massage and bodywork have been widely used and accepted in America. The changes in societal attitudes that took place during the 1960s included an interest in more natural ways of eating and of treating illness and injury. Since that time, there has been an increasing interest in the use of natural hands-on techniques for relieving bodily dysfunction.

Massage is becoming more accepted in the mainstream. About 17 percent of the adult U.S. population reported having massage in the past five years, with 8 percent in the past year. Massage is the most popular among individuals with some college education and college graduates.

On-site chair massage, which began in 1986, may be the fastest growing segment in the bodywork industry. Today there are more than ten thousand practitioners performing chair massage in the workplace. This trend indicates that a growing number of businesses are offering massage in the workplace because they recognize its value for productivity.

Another domain in which massage is becoming increasingly appreciated is sports. A growing number of teams are hiring massage therapists. Both trainers and athletes extol the benefits of massage and bodywork for enhancing performance and preventing muscular injury.

The knowledge of the preventive and healing value of touch is evidenced by the opening in 1991 of the Office of Alternative Medicine by the National Institutes of Health. Then, in 1997, Oxford Health Plan became the first health plan in the United States to offer an alternative medicine program, including massage, to its members.

The *Life* magazine article mentioned above discusses the increasing recognition of the power of touch in American society. The 1997 article states, "Massage has regained respectability in recent years and now enjoys unprecedented popularity. Some 25 million Americans make 60 million visits to 85,000 practitioners each year. Those numbers don't include employees of the growing number of institutions . . . that offer massage in the workplace. Or the children of the 10,000 parents who learn baby massage each year."

TOUCH RESEARCH INTERNATIONAL

The power of touch is so significant in human functioning that there is an internationally recognized institute devoted exclusively to the study of the power of touch. The Touch Research Institute at the University of Miami was created in 1991 by the University of Miami School of Medicine and is the world's first center for research on the impact of touch on human health and development. Because of the international impact of this institute, it has been renamed Touch Research International (TRI).

Touch Research International operates under the direction of Tiffany Field, Ph.D., a professor of psychology, pediatrics, and psychiatry at the University of Miami. The many studies performed by more than seventy scientists at TRI demonstrate the significant benefits of touch, in the form of massage, for both physical and mental health. Field has traveled the world spreading the word about the power of massage.

The exciting data on the benefits of massage point clearly to its value as a legitimate piece of the complex mosaic that comprises medical care today. According to the behavioral, physiological, and biochemical measures used to collect touch data at TRI, massage improves sleep patterns and reduces stress and depression.

TRI became famous after publishing research on premature babies, comparing those who received a regimen of massage with those who did not. The research demonstrated that the massaged population responded to therapeutic touch with weight gain, improved mental and motor development, and earlier discharge from the hospital. This last factor allows for parental touch of the newborn to occur earlier, which promotes bonding and healthy emotional development.

Although the research at TRI began with newborn babies, Field and her colleagues have researched the impact of massage on a wide range of populations including students, parents, depressed adolescents, and elders in nursing homes. Massage therapy has been shown to reduce anxiety and enhance EEG patterns of alertness in students. The decreased anxiety and increased alertness helped increase the speed and accuracy on math computations for the students who received fifteen minutes of chair massage two times per week for five weeks as compared with students who did not. Research shows that massage reduces "acting out" behavior, improves sleep patterns, and reduces depression in adolescents. Elders in nursing homes have a more positive outlook and feel better physically when receiving massage consistently.

The TRI research findings on the positive impact of massage on the health of individuals of all ages has been compelling. There are even ongoing investigations into prenatal massage. Research on the impact of massage continues to be funded because of the recognition of the role of massage in preventive medicine. As stated in the 1997 *Life* article on the power of touch, "And now science is confirming what we knew in our hearts: that . . . massage is medicine."

CHAPTER 2

Bodywork/Massage and Your Health

Having massage in your life is a health benefit. The positive effects on your health can be both immediate and long-lasting. Because the bulk of the research in this area has been done using massage, we will use *massage* as a generic term in this chapter without intending to omit any form of bodywork. All the massage and bodywork modalities have health benefits.

Although there are differences between approaches in the particular improvements or gains to be derived, there are also areas that overlap. In this chapter we want to introduce you to the overlap—the best reason to have massage in your life—for your health and feelings of well-being.

Bodywork and massage are not intended as a replacement for medication or medical treatments recommended by your doctor. However, the relaxation response induced by massage on both physical and mental levels triggers recuperative processes in the body and the mind. Combining conventional medical treatment with alternative approaches like massage can have a powerful impact on your health. The key element that empowers touch to affect our health is the constant interplay between body and mind.

THE RELATIONSHIP BETWEEN MIND AND BODY

Your body and your mind do not act independently of each other. The functioning of the body and the mind are closely intertwined and have an ongoing mutual impact. Their functioning is so reciprocal and interdependent that it is common for symptoms and illnesses to contain mental and emotional components as well as physical pain and discomfort. Wondering where the impact on health begins, with the body or with the mind, is like asking which came first, the chicken or the egg. Even though this is an unsolvable dilemma, let's examine each direction: body to mind and then mind to body.

Body Affects Mind

Your physical state affects your mental state and emotions. When a stimulus, either from the environment or from an internal source, impinges on the body, the mind is affected in the way we interpret, think, and feel. Positive bodily sensations produce positive mental states and feelings of well-being. Physical discomfort and pain can trigger a bleak outlook, obsessive thinking, anxiety, and mental fatigue.

Think about the impact of the body on the mind when you are ill. When you are physically debilitated or ill, you become focused on negative sensations in your body. Through this focus, your mental processes and emotions become negatively affected. For example, think about how difficult it is to concentrate or feel relaxed and happy (mind) when you are in pain or have the flu (body).

The nature of panic disorder provides a good illustration of the powerful impact of the body on the mind. Panic disorder, classified as a mental disorder, originates in the body. The mental and emotional experience of panic disorder can be triggered by a number of physical conditions, including mitral-valve prolapse, thyroid problems, and adrenal dysfunction. Let's take the case of mitral-valve prolapse, a relatively benign heart murmur that is genetic in origin. With this condition, the individual's mitral valve does not always close firmly as blood flows through it. Although the condition is not dangerous, it has associated symptoms that are unpleasant. When the valve flops or clicks, heart rate and blood pressure elevate slightly, making the person feel wired. These changes occur without warning. Not realizing that the changes are purely physical and harmless, the individual experiencing them begins to worry about the increased heart rate and agitated feeling. The anxiety causes the heart to pound even faster. These symptoms are accompanied by sweatiness, dizziness, and more anxiety, escalating to a full-blown panic attack with feelings of impending doom and fears of going crazy or dying.

Because the individual might be anywhere when the mitral valve works improperly, the anxiety and panic become associated with a variety of locations, like the supermarket, workplace, or car. Panic disorder can lead to agoraphobia, avoidance of going places, and restriction of one's life. And it all begins with a harmless leaky valve.

Mind Affects Body

The reciprocal also holds. Your mental state and emotions affect your physical well-being. When you feel stressed, anxious, or depressed (mind) for a prolonged period, you are likely to suffer physically (body) for a number of reasons. These include the tendency to neglect your own physical needs when you are preoccupied, tense, and unhappy; an increase in the secretion of chemicals that impairs the optimal functioning of your bodily systems; and blockages in the flow of natural healing energy.

When we feel confident and clearheaded, we allow our bodies to relax and function more effectively. When negative or fearful thoughts are spinning around in our minds, our bodies tense up.

There are hundreds of research studies that demonstrate the impact of the mind on the body. For example, people under hypnosis are able to change physiological processes in their bodies by imagining the changes or by mentally directing their bodies to make changes. Individuals have used hypnosis and mental imagery for many years to reduce skin rashes, to break habits like smoking, and to enhance athletic performance. Such results demonstrate the power of the mind on the functioning of the body.

Regardless of the origin of the discomfort—the body or the mind— a spiraling cycle can easily develop. It is the combination of mental and physical tension and chronic discomfort fueled by the negative exchanges between body and mind that is known as stress. Stress not only *feels* bad, it *is* bad for you.

STRESS AND YOUR HEALTH

The relationship between stress and illness is well documented and widely accepted. It has been estimated that up to 90 percent of visits to primary care physicians are associated with stress-related complaints. The most common symptoms reported include physical fatigue, emotional exhaustion, head-aches, backaches, neck pain, eyestrain, poor concentration, anxiety, depression, irritable bowel, stomach pain and discomfort, and high blood pressure. Stress can be a big factor in triggering and maintaining any of these problems.

Stress begins with a stressor. Everyone is exposed to stressors throughout the day. A *stressor* is an event over which you have no control and which has the potential to trigger a stress reaction with physical, mental, and emotional components. Examples of stressors include your car not starting in the morning when you are late for an appointment or your boss denying you a personal day. Big or small, such events can trigger negative thoughts and physical tension. As the mental and physical reactions to external stressors grow in intensity through the activity in the mind-body feedback loop, we begin to experience stress.

Stress makes all the systems of the body work harder and less efficiently, which is what makes us prone to illness and dysfunction. The mental tension triggered by the events of everyday life quickly signals the brain to tense your muscles through the release of stress hormones from the adrenal glands. These stress hormones cause your blood vessels to constrict and reduce circulation. As a result, your heart works harder, your breathing becomes more rapid and shallow, and your digestive system slows down.

In fact, nearly all bodily systems are affected negatively by stress. The ripple effect of this sluggishness of bodily systems leaves the cells of the body and brain deprived of oxygen and other nutrients. Waste products accumulate without being eliminated efficiently from body tissue. The result is a weakened internal environment and mental and emotional exhaustion. In this condition, the body cannot easily prevent and fight disease.

There are actually stress hormones that can literally kill brain cells in the hippocampus, a structure in the brain critical to learning and memory. Stress can be a causal factor in migraine headaches, chronic pain, high blood pressure, heart disease, peptic ulcers, depression, and other disorders.

MASSAGE CAN BREAK THE STRESS CYCLE

The key mechanism through which massage improves health is stress reduction. One thread running through the various approaches to massage and bodywork is the guiding principle that too much stress suppresses your immune system, threatening your health and well-being. The touch provided in massage and bodywork can break this potentially devastating stress cycle.

Massage Reduces Stress

Research has shown that massage can provide relief from both the physical and mental symptoms of stress. In numerous publications, including *Prevention* magazine (December 1990), massage is referred to as a proven technique for the reduction of both physical and mental stress. If stress causes illness and massage reduces stress, then it logically follows that massage can be used as a legitimate preventive and healing adjunct to medical treatments.

Scientific studies conducted at Touch Research International demonstrate the relationship between massage and stress reduction by measuring changes in physiological and biochemical indicators before and after massage. Stress reduction via massage has been proven by massage receivers' decreased pulse rates, lower levels of the stress hormones (cortisol and norepinephrine), and more efficient functioning of neurotransmitters, including dopamine.

Therapeutic, Nurturing Touch Sends
Positive Messages to the Brain

Massage has this powerful positive impact because the soothing physical sensations produced by these professional hands-on procedures feed back to the brain and reduce mental stress. Once mental stress is reduced, the brain sends signals to the adrenal glands to stop releasing stress hormones and signals the muscles to unwind. This feedback loop between the mental and physical manifestations of stress explains why massaging one area of the body can produce a feeling of relaxation throughout the entire body.

Massage Reduces Stress and Improves Health by Promoting Circulation

Massage also relieves both physical and mental stress by improving circulation. In massage, the practitioner's strokes relax the tense muscles that may have interfered with efficient blood flow. The direction and rhythm of the strokes encourage blood to flow through the veins and back toward the heart. When your circulatory system is working optimally, sufficient oxygen and nutrients will be able to reach and nourish the cells throughout your body.

In addition to improving blood circulation, the benefits of massage extend to improving the flow of lymph through the lymphatic system, which rids the blood and body tissues of toxins and waste products. When the lymphatic system becomes constricted and inefficient, the accumulating waste products take the body out of a balanced state and create physical stress, discomfort, and eventually health problems. When your blood is flowing freely through arteries and veins and your lymph is circulating properly, you experience renewed energy. Your immune system functions more effectively to prevent disease and to heal the body from illness and injury.

Massage Reduces Stress by Triggering the Release of Endorphins

The touch of massage can reduce stress and produce feelings of well-being by triggering the release of endorphins by the brain. Research has shown that endorphin levels increase with the application of massage. Endorphins are considered such potent painkillers that they are known as natural opiates. An increase in endorphin production leads to a more pleasurable body state, a higher energy level, and greater physical and mental endurance. Stronger, ongoing touch can have a more lasting impact.

Massage Reduces Stress by Relieving Physical Symptoms

Massage can provide relief from the pain and soreness of muscle tension. The massage and bodywork modalities vary in their techniques of addressing tension and pain. The approaches are based on different theories of the origin of pain and how to treat pain symptoms. What they have in common is the goal of alleviating chronic physical symptoms, which also relieves chronic stress.

CONTRAINDICATIONS

In your decision process regarding massage and bodywork, it is important that you consider any possible contraindications. A contraindication is a condition that makes using a particular treatment inadvisable. For example, being pregnant may make it inadvisable for you to take certain medications or be exposed to certain medical procedures. Reasons for postponing massage and bodywork include having a fever or an acute infectious disease. Specific contraindications vary from one modality to another. The massage therapist or bodywork practitioner will ask you questions to rule out contraindications. Sometimes only certain areas of the body will be contraindicated, for example, a rash on your arm or leg might mean avoiding lubrication or pressure on those areas. Always consult your physician if you are unsure. For most people, massage is a safe, beneficial piece of the fabric of health care.

THINK ABOUT YOUR HEALTH GOALS

Has your doctor recommended that you reduce and stabilize your high blood pressure? Do you have an old sports injury that still bothers you? Are you seeking relief from muscle spasms, soreness, or tension? Do you want to improve your flexibility and move more easily? Are you trying to get your energy back? Is it better skin tone you are after? Do you want to improve the quality of your sleep? Is your goal to alleviate anxiety or depression? Or do you feel okay but want increased vitality or deeper feelings of well-being?

There are many different massage and bodywork approaches that can help you achieve one or more of your health goals. That is why we consider this book a guide to improving your physical and mental health through the healing power of touch.

CHAPTER 3

The Giver/Receiver Relationship

Bodywork and massage are hands-on processes of healing that involve two individuals: one who gives the treatment and one who receives the treatment. *Giver* and *receiver* are broad terms borrowed from the Eastern philosophy of massage. In some modalities, givers call themselves massage therapists; in others, bodywork practitioners; and in still others, teachers. In Therapeutic Touch, the giver is referred to as a healer and the receiver as a healee. In most modalities, however, receivers are considered clients.

GIVING

What is given? Most often, what is given is information and systematic therapeutic touch. In some modalities, the touch is deeper than in others. Some approaches are more oriented toward relaxation, whereas others focus more on movement or integration of the body as a whole entity. In some modalities, the giver's role is to impart positive energy through the hands to the body of the receiver.

Regardless of the specific techniques of giving, in order to give effectively, the giver must establish trust with the receiver. Establishing trust involves providing the receiver with a nonthreatening, accepting attitude and environment and making it clear that the receiver's feelings of comfort and safety are paramount.

RECEIVING

What is received? The receiver gets information, and the receiver experiences the nurturing impact of touch, feelings of well-being, and healing on many levels. There is a wide variety of massage and bodywork modalities. Each one offers a different path to healing.

In order to receive effectively, the receiver must be willing to trust the giver. He or she must be able to speak openly to the giver regarding comfort, feelings of safety, concerns, and goals at any point during treatment. As the receiver, you have the right to terminate treatment before the session is over without the threat of disapproval from the giver.

As a receiver, you may be more passive or more active, depending on your personality and on the parameters of the chosen modality. Regardless of modality, it is always appropriate to ask questions and make sure you are comfortable with the giver and the environment.

BOUNDARIES IN PROFESSIONAL MASSAGE

The roles of giver and receiver should not get blurred. Even though in certain modalities the receiver plays an active and communicative role during treatment, the receiver remains in the receiver role, and the giver remains in the giver role. There can be no overlap in the roles of giver and receiver. It is the clear boundary between giver and receiver in professional massage that creates safety for both the professional and the client.

Even though giving and receiving are intimate experiences because of the hands-on nature of the therapies, the intimacy is not intended to be sexual in nature. For the receiver, the intimacy takes the form of being a willing receiver, allowing oneself to relax and be open to the process of receiving. Being touched during massage feels good as physical and mental tension are relieved for the receiver, who is appropriately more self-absorbed than involved with the giver of the service. For the giver, the intimacy takes the clinical form of constantly assessing the feedback from the receiver's muscles or body energy and becoming familiar with the receiver's needs so that these needs can be addressed within the boundaries of professional practice.

Professional massage and bodywork are not supposed to be a sexual experience for either the giver or the receiver and need not be a threat to you or your spouse. Bodywork and massage are widely accepted forms of treatment for a variety of health-related problems. Practitioners are trained in ethical conduct and professionalism. Sex has no place in professional massage and bodywork. There is no need to give the relationship a sexual connotation, unless, of course, one of you is doing something inappropriate. If you feel uncomfortable during treatment, you can stop the session at once. You have the option of finding another practitioner just as you do when you engage a doctor, a lawyer, or any other helping professional.

Givers are trained to be aware of and sensitive to the receiver's apprehensions. Receivers are informed that they can leave on any garments they wish for massage. Some bodywork modalities require little or no disrobing.

In traditional massage, the client is carefully draped, with modesty protected at all times. Massage therapists do not touch breasts or genitals. If there are any other parts of your body that you do not want touched, let the massage therapist know, and your wishes should be respected.

Boundaries are set by the giver as well. They include not dating or engaging in sexual conduct or even socializing with the receiver. Boundaries must be set regarding scheduling so that the client does not infringe on the giver's personal life by demanding immediate massages. Time boundaries must also be set; it cannot be expected that the giver will go overtime without compensation. The receiver is expected to be timely for appointments so that the giver can keep his or her schedule intact.

In addition, the giver must clearly define the scope of the modality to be performed. For example, it would be inappropriate to claim that Swedish massage alleviates trigger points or that neuromuscular therapy cures arthritis.

COMMUNICATION BETWEEN GIVER AND RECEIVER

Your first communication will most likely be over the phone, when you arrange the initial session. This first contact gives you the opportunity to get an impression of the giver and to ask questions about the treatment and express any concerns you might have, including how to prepare for the session.

Questions to Ask

- How long have you been practicing massage or bodywork?
- Where were you trained?
- What are your credentials?
- Are you a member of the American Massage Therapy Association (AMTA) or any other professional associations?

    ❧ Do you accept insurance?

    ❧ What is your fee structure? Do you accept checks? Credit cards?

    ❧ Do I have to do anything special to prepare for the massage (or bodywork)?

    ❧ Do you use oil or cream?

    ❧ Will I have to remove my clothing?

    ❧ How long is the session?

Request for Receiver's History

Once you arrive for your session, the giver will greet you and ask you—orally or in writing or both—some questions about your health history and the state of your body. It is important to disclose the necessary information. The purpose of the questions is to determine your needs and whether there are contraindications to your receiving in that modality. The amount of assessment after this point depends on the modality. For example, in the case of Swedish massage, the assessment work is brief, whereas in the myofascial release and neuromuscular modalities, which address deeper and more complex issues, the assessment phase is longer and requires more in-depth communication between giver and receiver.

Typical Questions Asked by the Giver

    ❧ How did you hear about me?

    ❧ What would you like to get from this massage (or bodywork)?

    ❧ Have you had massage (or bodywork) before? What was your experience like?

    ❧ What types of modalities have you received?

    ❧ What are your major areas of concern?

    ❧ Are there any areas you would like me to avoid?

The amount and nature of verbal exchange during treatment depends on the type of massage or bodywork modality and the personalities of receiver and giver. Some approaches (e.g., Hellerwork) entail a series of sessions, and communication would be a vital part of the process. However, there are forms of massage which can be undertaken as onetime, occasional, or even frequent sessions in which little communication is necessary. It is okay to enjoy a massage and say nothing at all throughout the experience.

Confidential Case History

The giver may ask the receiver to complete a confidential case history form before treatment begins. The purpose of collecting this information is to uncover any contraindications and determine an effective course of treatment. The following is an example of a format for a confidential case history:

Name: _____

Address: _____

Home phone: _____

Work phone: _____

Age: _____ Date of birth: _____ M/F: _____

Marital status: _____ Number of children: _____

Occupation: _____

How did you hear about us? _____

Who is responsible for payment? _____

Have you had massage before? _____

Where and by whom? _____

_____

What is your major area of pain or concern? _____

_____

When did you first notice it? _____

What brought it on? _____

What activities aggravate it? _____

Is this condition getting better or worse? _____

Does it interfere with work? _____

Sleep? _____   Recreation? _____

What have you done so far to get relief? _____

_____

Has there been a medical exam? _____

Diagnosis? _____

X rays? _____   Blood work? _____

What was the diagnosis? _____

_____

By whom? _____

Other areas of pain or concern? _____

_____

Are you presently under a doctor's care? _____

If so, for what condition(s)? _____

Name of physician: _____

Phone: _____

List any medications you are currently taking: _____

_____

List previous operation: _____

Previous broken bones: _____

Previous accidents or injuries: _____

_____

The confidential case history may also ask you to check off on a provided list symptoms and conditions that pertain to you.

PAYMENT METHOD

Payment is generally required at the time treatment is given unless a prepaid package of massages or a gift certificate was previously purchased or another arrangement was agreed on. In some states, certain insurance companies will make direct payment to the massage therapist or will provide the receiver with reimbursement. Some massage therapists make house calls for an additional fee.

Massage therapists will always accept cash, almost always accept checks, and may be equipped to accept certain credit cards. In some modalities in which bodywork is given in a set series of sessions, the method and timing of payment will be specified in advance. The cost of massage and bodywork will vary depending on modality, length of session, setting, and geographical location.

CHOOSING A GIVER

Your first task before choosing a giver is to choose the modalities that you feel would best address your needs. The next chapter lists the modalities included in this book. The remainder of the book is devoted to giving you a description and flavor of nineteen modalities. In appendix B, you will be provided with resources that will lead you to trained massage therapists and bodywork practitioners of the modalities described.

In addition to checking out training and credentials, it is also important that you feel comfortable and welcomed by the giver you select. Remember that you will be the receiver. Trust your intuition when making your choice.

CHAPTER 4

Bodywork and Massage Modalities

The *Bodywork and Massage Sourcebook* is designed to provide you with information on a wide variety of modalities that use the power of touch for the purpose of enhancing your feelings of well-being and improving your physical and mental health. In addition to making you feel good, the various massage and bodywork modalities can be undertaken in order to address a variety of health issues. We view massage and bodywork as useful adjuncts to traditional medical treatment, not as substitute methods.

DEFINING BODYWORK AND MASSAGE

Although the terms *bodywork* and *massage* sometimes overlap, there are certain distinctions. All forms of massage fall under the category of bodywork, but there are other forms of bodywork that are not considered massage.

Massage and bodywork are both hands-on practices that involve tactile manipulation of muscles and muscle tissue. Unlike massage, however,
bodywork also addresses other issues and aspects of human functioning.

The intensity of the practitioner's touch varies in both massage and
bodywork from light strokes to deep-tissue work, depending on the modality and the goals. In the bodywork modalities based on energy-field theory,
there is no direct contact with the skin for all or for part of the session.

Some of the areas addressed by bodywork, rather than massage alone,
include energy forces, bodily posture, the structural integrity of the body,
fluidity of bodily movement, and emotional release. Not all forms of bodywork address all of these areas. You can decide as you read about the modalities included in this sourcebook what your needs and desires are and which
massage or bodywork modalities would best suit your current needs.
Massage and bodywork can have a major impact on how you feel, no matter whether the touch is gentle or deep or whether the work focuses on your
anatomy or on your energy.

MANY GOOD OPTIONS

There are at least fifty separate bodywork and massage modalities. We
selected nineteen modalities that are well-known and span the categories
and types of bodywork and massage available. Our goal in the selection was
to provide you with information about modalities that are representative of
a wide range of choices you can make.

Some of the modalities described have their roots in Eastern philosophy and practice; others are Western in origin; still others are hybrids. Some
modalities focus on deep-tissue work; others involve lighter, gentler touch.

Some forms of massage are designed to promote relaxation, whereas others are more specifically therapeutic in nature. Certain forms of bodywork focus on somatic education, movement, and posture, whereas others involve healing through unblocking energy. Some of the modalities combine various elements of touch, relaxation, healing, and education. The particular origins and focus of each modality will be explained in the chapter that pertains to that specific modality.

THE MODALITIES

The following bodywork and massage modalities are covered in this book:

- Swedish massage
- Infant massage
- Sports massage
- Geriatric massage
- Myofascial release
- Neuromuscular therapy
- Shiatsu
- Reflexology
- Trager Approach
- Manual lymph drainage
- Craniosacral therapy
- Rosen Method
- Rolfing
- Hellerwork
- Alexander Technique
- Feldenkrais Method
- Reiki
- Polarity Therapy
- Therapeutic Touch

THE COST OF BODYWORK/MASSAGE

The cost of bodywork and massage varies widely depending on the modality, the setting in which it is received, geographical area, length of session, and the practitioner. For example, you might pay as little as twenty-five dollars for a one-hour Swedish massage at a clinic associated with a massage school, and as much as one hundred dollars for the same service at a day spa. The more typical cost for this service will fall somewhere in between. The range in cost will be just as varied for receiving other modalities.

A growing number of health insurance plans consider massage and other forms of bodywork valid forms of treatment for a variety of disorders, and there are clinics and practitioners who work for affordable fees.

Many schools that train massage therapists run a massage clinic in which the students being trained provide massage under supervision of qualified massage therapists to the public at reasonable rates. Rates for senior citizens are even lower at many clinics. For specific information on rates in the variety of settings that provide bodywork and massage, you would have to contact the school, clinic, practitioner, or spa directly.

Massaging the Stress Away

Swedish Massage

Infant Massage

Sports Massage

Geriatric Massage

Myofascial Release

Swedish massage is the most familiar modality, and that is where we will begin. After a description of the history, experience, and benefits of Swedish massage, you will be introduced to its adaptation for special populations: infants and children, athletes, and aging adults. Myofascial release, which focuses on the fascia, is a more recently developed and deeper form of massage than Swedish and its derivatives.

CHAPTER 5

Swedish Massage

Swedish massage is the most popular and well-known massage modality in the United States and Europe. People thinking of getting a massage for the first time usually opt for a Swedish massage. A good Swedish massage is an extremely enjoyable experience. In addition, this traditional Western form of massage promotes health and relaxation by relieving muscle tension and improving circulation. The American Massage Therapy Association describes Swedish massage as a system of long strokes, kneading, and friction techniques on the more superficial layers of the muscles, combined with active and passive movements of the joints.

Many people have experienced massage only on a cruise or at a spa. Swedish massage is the most prevalent form of massage offered on vacations because of its relaxing, mellowing impact. Unfortunately, too many people attend to their bodily needs only when on vacation and neglect themselves during nonvacation time, when stress is more common. We make excuses like, "I'm too busy to get a massage." If you perceive your life this way, then you are a good candidate for a Swedish massage.

HISTORY OF SWEDISH MASSAGE

Swedish massage was developed by Per Henrik Ling. Ling was born in Sweden in 1776. As a young man he earned a degree in divinity. Later, he became a physiologist and a fencing master. He also studied medicine and wrote poetry. From an early age, Ling suffered from rheumatoid arthritis. Combining his diverse skills and knowledge of blood circulation with information he gathered while seeking pain relief, Ling developed a system of massage and gymnastic movement exercises that not only cured his arthritis but also became legendary.

Ling's system of massage and active and passive movements became known as the Ling System or the Swedish Movement Treatment. In 1813, a school known as the Royal Swedish Central Institute was established in Stockholm by the Swedish government, and Ling was named the president of the institute. Although the traditional medical establishment initially rejected Ling's form of treatment, the acceptance of the Ling System was widespread because of its effectiveness. People came to Stockholm from the United States to learn the Ling System. When Ling died in 1839, his students in Europe made his methods known throughout the world. Over time, the original Ling System evolved into Swedish massage as it is practiced today.

THE STROKES OF SWEDISH MASSAGE

The strokes used in Swedish massage are designed to relieve muscle tension. The muscles throughout your body begin to systematically relax with the rhythm of the massage. As your muscles relax, your brain will receive signals to trigger the release of chemicals that reduce stress and produce feelings of well-being.

There are five classic strokes that originated with Swedish massage (Table 5.1). The strokes are made with the massage therapist's hands in the direction of blood flow toward the heart. Stroking the soft tissue of the body in this direction promotes blood circulation, which is one of the goals and benefits of Swedish massage.

TABLE 5.1   CLASSIC STROKES OF SWEDISH MASSAGE

Stroke	Qualities
Effleurage	Light, gentle gliding strokes; ranges from superficial to deep; applied in the direction of the heart
Petrissage	Usually follows effleurage; kneading the muscles like dough; improves circulation of nutrients and elimination of wastes
Friction	Compression movements; rubbing; deeper than effleurage and petrissage; releases deeper layers of tension and promotes circulation
Tapotement	Tapping; percussive movements; good for muscle spasms
Vibration	Gentle shaking of the body; can be stimulating or relaxing depending on duration

Any combination or all of the five strokes may be used in one Swedish massage session. It is the way these strokes are applied and combined that tailors the massage to the client's needs. The combination, depth, and duration of massage movements is determined by the massage therapist, who is constantly in tune with the receiver's physical and verbal responses. The therapist uses this feedback to plan the massage and to make adjustments during the course of the massage.

Differences in the way the strokes are applied produce differences in outcome. For example, when Swedish massage strokes are applied slowly, the massage can make you feel sleepy, whereas when the strokes are applied more rapidly and with deeper pressure, the massage can be invigorating and energizing.

SETTINGS FOR RECEIVING SWEDISH MASSAGE

Swedish massage is the most widely available form of massage and can be received in a variety of settings. As mentioned before, many individuals experience Swedish massage for the first time while on vacation at a resort or spa or on a cruise ship. Swedish massage is offered at day spas all over the country. Many gyms and health clubs now offer Swedish massage, some with discounted rates for members. You can also receive Swedish massage from students and teachers at clinics that are associated with massage therapy schools. Many massage therapists in private practice offer Swedish massage at their offices. Some massage therapists make home visits for an additional fee and bring the massage table and supplies with them.

THE EXPERIENCE OF SWEDISH MASSAGE

During Swedish massage, the receiver lies under a towel or sheet on a comfortable, padded massage therapy table. The best way to receive Swedish massage is with your body unclothed. Swedish massage therapists are trained to respect their clients' privacy and to use draping techniques that protect the clients' genitals and breasts from being exposed or touched. However, if you are uncomfortable being completely unclothed under the sheet, you may wear minimal clothing (e.g., underpants), and still reap the benefits of Swedish massage.

History Taking

Before the massage begins, the massage therapist will ask you about past injuries, surgeries, and tender, sensitive, or sore areas of your body. Your answers to these questions will determine if you have any contraindications. These include (but are not limited to) pregnancy in the first trimester, running a recent fever, active infection, vomiting, nausea, diarrhea, bleeding, and conditions that can lead to blood clotting.

Before the massage begins, you can discuss with the therapist what you hope to gain from it. The massage therapist can adjust the depth, duration, and combination of strokes, which will influence whether you feel mellow or invigorated after the massage. It is also important that you discuss with the massage therapist whether any parts of your body are sensitive to touch. For example, you might want to tell the therapist in advance if your feet are ticklish. All the information you provide will guide the massage therapist in meeting your needs.

Disrobing

After your discussion, the therapist will leave you alone to disrobe and get on the table under the sheet. You will have been instructed either to lie on your back or to lie on your stomach with your head in a face cradle, an adjustable attachment to the table which comfortably houses your face and supports your head when you are lying facedown during Swedish massage. It is more likely that you will be asked to start by lying on your back. While waiting for the massage therapist to return, you can begin to relax your body and mind by focusing your attention on your breathing, which should be slow and even. The massage therapist will knock gently on the door before entering.

The Massage

Swedish massage is a whole body massage. You are free to indicate to the massage therapist at any time any areas where you prefer lighter touch, deeper touch, or no touch. Massage oil or lotion is used to lubricate the body. The lubrication reduces the friction of the strokes, allowing for sufficient pressure to alleviate muscle tension. If you have an allergy to a particular type of oil or lotion or if you prefer light lubrication, you should share this information with the massage therapist. Your right to share information and communicate about your needs is part of the benefit of Swedish massage.

The massage therapist will then apply a combination of the strokes of Swedish massage (effleurage, petrissage, friction, tapotement, and vibration) at a depth of touch and duration best suited to your body and to your stated wishes. Techniques from other massage and bodywork modalities may be interwoven with the classic strokes of Swedish massage. A good eclectic massage therapist knows how to artfully combine a foundation of classic

Swedish massage with selected techniques from other modalities and create a cohesive whole tailored to the needs of each individual client.

After working on one side of your body for about half an hour, the massage therapist will ask you to turn over and will then work on the other side of your body for about the same amount of time.

On either or both sides of your body, the massage therapist might suggest and initiate joint movements. These are gentle stretches and rotations designed to loosen tight joints. These assisted movements may be active or passive. As the joint movements progress, they gently relieve tightness and soreness and enhance your range of motion.

"Relax a Few Minutes Before Getting Up"

Many Swedish massage therapists use these words after they have completed the massage. Then they leave you alone in the room for a few minutes. Would you take this opportunity to relax for a few minutes before getting up, as suggested, or bolt up and get dressed?

It is worth taking advantage of the opportunity to remain on the table in a relaxed state for a few minutes. Letting your body and mind appreciate the aftermath of the massage helps reinforce the feelings of well-being achieved during the massage. Absorbing the full impact of the massage will help you remember how to re-create those good feelings later in the day, even later in the week, when stressors impinge on you.

PHYSICAL AND EMOTIONAL BENEFITS

Swedish massage is designed to produce feelings of well-being on both the physical and emotional levels. Beyond helping you feel good, Swedish massage has real physical and emotional benefits.

Swedish massage helps the body eliminate toxins, improves blood and lymph circulation, increases range of motion in the joints, and alleviates muscle tension and soreness. It promotes physical relaxation and reduces pain through the release of endorphins, the body's natural opiates.

The reduction in muscular tension goes hand in hand with positive mental health outcomes including decreased anxiety and depression, improved ability to concentrate, and deeper states of relaxation. Swedish massage relieves mental and physical fatigue and reduces stress on both superficial and deep levels. Swedish massage helps people overcome sleep difficulties, including falling asleep and staying asleep throughout the night.

Research has shown that Swedish massage can relieve asthma in children. In a 1995 study at Brown University, mothers gave their asthmatic children twenty-minute massages every evening at bedtime for one month. The data revealed that these children had fewer asthma attacks and were able to breathe better based on daily peak air-flow readings when compared with asthmatic children who received no massage. An additional benefit was that the children's mood improved, their levels of the stress hormone cortisol decreased, and both the children's and mothers' anxiety decreased.

Swedish massage is a modality that benefits people of all ages, from newborns to the geriatric population. Massage studies at Touch Research International have demonstrated that massage helps premature babies thrive, reduces anxiety and depression in children and adolescents, and lowers depression, stress, and loneliness in elders. These conclusions are based not only on the participants' subjective experience of increased feelings of well-being but also on the positive physiological and biochemical changes after massage, including lower levels of stress hormones.

Benefits of Swedish Massage

Enhanced feelings of well-being on both the physical and emotional levels.

Reduction in the physical and mental components of stress.

Less muscle tension and soreness.

Relief of tension and migraine headaches.

More effective elimination of toxins.

Improved blood and lymph circulation.

Lower blood pressure.

Increased range of motion in the joints.

Enhanced flexibility.

Higher levels of endorphins.

Less anxiety.

Relief from depression.

Improved ability to concentrate.

Relief from mental and physical fatigue.

Less stress on superficial and deep levels.

Less trouble sleeping.

It can be used by people of all ages, from newborns to the geriatric population.

Relief from asthma symptoms.

SELECTING A SWEDISH MASSAGE THERAPIST

Some people do a little research before selecting a massage therapist. They may consult a friend who receives massage or read about Swedish massage. Other people decide to get a massage on impulse, because they've happened to see a massage therapist's signboard or advertisement. Regardless of how you make your choice, it is important to consider the therapist's training and credentials.

There is little consistency in institutional and state requirements concerning the training of massage therapists, and some states still have no licensure for massage therapy. The organization that holds the field of massage therapy up to a consistently high standard is the American Massage Therapy Association. To be approved by the AMTA, schools must provide a program that includes five hundred hours of training; a combination of basic courses in anatomy, physiology, and pathology; and applied coursework and practice in massage therapy. Some massage therapists are further credentialed by having passed a national exam given by the National Certification Board for Therapeutic Massage and Bodywork.

CHAPTER 6

Infant Massage

The warm, nurturing, aquatic environment of the mother's womb is complete and soothing to the unborn child. Through the process of birth, the baby loses the security and perfection of the fetal environment. Loving touch can ease the transition. Gentle, consistent touch from the very beginning of the child's life is key to providing a nurturing foundation. Healthy physical and emotional development is grounded in the caring environment provided during infancy.

THE POWER OF TOUCH FOR BABIES

For babies, the first communications received are through the skin. The skin is the largest organ in the body with the greatest number of receptor cells. The sense of touch develops in humans before the more distal senses of hearing and seeing. Thus, the hands of the baby's caregivers are a big part of the baby's world.

Among the many things that the caregiver's hands can do for the baby, nurturing touch is one of the most important. Touch messages stimulate the nervous system and brain in an infant just as they do in an adult. The difference is that the infant's brain and nervous system are still forming. Thus, the information received early in life becomes an actual part of the internal systems of the growing infant. All of the child's future experiences will be interpreted by the brain and the brain's chemistry according to the patterns established by early signals, including touch signals, to the brain and nervous system.

Touch and Survival

Tactile stimulation from the beginning of life is necessary not only for healthy development but also for survival. Being touched is a physical requirement for stimulating the infant's nervous system. Babies who are fed but never touched will fail to thrive and eventually die from the lack of tactile stimulation. Although most infants receive sufficient touch early in life to survive, many troubled children and adults grew up in households where nurturing touch was rarely seen or personally experienced.

Infant massage enhances the amount and quality of touch the baby receives. There exists substantial evidence that the touch provided in infant massage promotes the health and well-being of full-term babies and premature babies. The provider of massage to the infant, generally a parent or grandparent, benefits as well.

Touch and Bonding

Both research and common sense indicate that touching promotes bonding between parent and baby. Bonding is the foundation of the lifelong love and attachment between parent and child. Infant massage provides a wonderful structured time for parent and child to communicate on a deeper level.

Feelings of security and safety promoted by nurturing touch help infants learn to trust their caregivers and themselves. Learning to trust in infancy leads to self-confidence and self-esteem in childhood and adolescence, critical factors in determining quality of life in adulthood. Once trust and healthy bonding are established, the growing child feels confident enough to explore, create, achieve, develop a sense of identity, and bond with others.

RESEARCH SHOWS BENEFITS OF INFANT MASSAGE

Infant massage has been intensively researched in the scientific community since the 1970s. The first studies targeted premature babies as the subjects. Since then, healthy babies and mothers have been studied as well.

Premature Babies Make Progress with Massage

In 1975, a doctoral dissertation at the University of Texas demonstrated the powerful benefits of massage for thirty premature babies. The massaged premature babies showed better development of their nervous systems as compared with nonmassaged babies. The specific, measurable changes in the brain and nervous system included an increase in myelin, a substance that coats certain neurons and facilitates neural transmission, and an increase in the output of the hypothalamus, the arousal center of the brain.

The massaged babies also had a higher output of somatotrophin, a growth hormone that promotes weight gain, a critical factor in the well-being of premature babies.

Research performed by Tiffany Field, Ph.D., and her colleagues from the 1980s through the present has verified the value of massage for infants. In a seminal study in 1986, when infants born premature of crack-addicted mothers were not developing well and were massaged, the results were remarkable. When these babies were massaged for fifteen minutes three times a day, they gained weight 47 percent faster than such babies who were not massaged, even though the food intake was the same. The massaged babies simply developed better than those not massaged. The massaged babies required shorter hospital stays by six days than the nonmassaged babies, resulting in a significant cost savings. Eight months later, the massaged babies continued to demonstrate better mental and motor development than the nonmassaged babies and also had maintained their weight advantage.

Infant massage was used to promote the health and growth of the history-making septuplets born in the United States in 1997. Premature babies who receive consistent massage achieve higher scores on the Brazelton Scales, which measure habituation to stimuli, orientation, motor activity, and regulation of internal bodily states. Being able to regulate your internal state and keep your body in harmony contributes to maintaining health throughout your life span.

Massage Helps Babies with Health Problems

In a recent series of studies on the health impact of massage on the pediatric population, Field and her colleagues at Touch Research International had parents gently massage their babies for fifteen to twenty minutes a night just before bedtime over a period of thirty days. Massaged children with juvenile diabetes had lower blood-sugar levels than those not massaged. Massaged children with asthma showed an immediate decrease in anxiety and stress-hormone levels, after which their peak air-flow and pulmonary functions improved as compared with asthmatic children not massaged. Massage also reduced skin rashes and sleep difficulties in children. Field believes that these results confirm that systematic, nurturing touch in the form of massage triggers physiological changes that facilitate the growth and development of infants and children.

Infant massage has been used to relax the muscles of physically handicapped babies. The relaxation, and perhaps the facilitation of the mind-body connection, helped these children improve their functioning.

Infant Massage Helps Depressed Mothers and Their Babies

Field's research also addresses the impact of infant massage on the giver. As you might anticipate, providing your baby with massage makes you feel good. Research shows that massaging your baby reduces stress for both you and your baby.

It is estimated that during pregnancy 10 to 12 percent of expectant mothers suffer from chronic depression. Between 25 to 30 percent of mothers experience postpartum depression during the first three months after delivery. According to Field, babies mirror the emotions of their primary caregiver, including the symptoms of depression. Infants born to depressed mothers have elevated stress hormones, show little facial expression, have loss of appetite, and have poor sleep. If left untreated, these depressed newborns will grow into depressed infants and children who, if not treated, will grow into depressed adolescents and adults.

How can you treat depression in a newborn or an infant? The answer is through the touch provided by infant massage. If a depressed mother is willing to break through the depression barrier for the sake of avoiding or alleviating depression in her infant, she will reap the rewards of having helped her child and, in addition, feel better herself.

Research has shown that infant massage helps both depressed mothers and babies. Depressed mothers who performed infant massage daily for two weeks played more with their infant and perceived their babies as easier to soothe. They also felt more empowered because they played a role in their babies' increased vocalizations, more organized sleep, and decreased fussiness. When babies were massaged for six weeks, they cried less, had better sleep patterns, were more responsive to people, and showed a decrease in stress hormones. The results of this research has positive implications for the use of infant massage to promote better parenting attitudes and skills.

Massage Is Good for Healthy Babies and Their Parents

Massage benefits healthy babies and children as well as those with health and stress-related problems. Massage is relaxing for both baby and parent and promotes bonding. The touch of massage helps maintain the elastic quality of your baby's muscles and skin and teaches your baby how to relax, whether in motion or at rest.

Massage prepares the baby's body for sitting, standing, and walking by promoting the baby's strength, motor coordination, and self-confidence. Massage in infancy may prevent some of the structural integration problems and dysfunctional movement patterns that so many adults develop from poor early habits.

Benefits of Infant Massage

Relaxation of both baby and parent.

Less stress for both baby and parent.

Closer parent-child bonding.

Babies learn how to relax both when in motion and when at rest.

The elastic quality of your baby's muscles and skin is maintained.

Increased strength, motor coordination, and self-confidence.

Preparation for sitting, standing, and walking.

Improved circulation, respiration, digestion, and elimination.

Stimulation of the baby's nervous system and immune system.

Better sleep patterns.

Less colic.

Comfort during illness or injury or when facing a medical procedure.

Relief from aches, fever, and congestion.

Giver can check baby's body for areas of discomfort or bruises.

Faster weight gain and developmental progress in premature babies.

Symptom relief for children with asthma, physical disabilities, or juvenile diabetes.

Infant massage improves circulation, respiration, digestion, and elimination in healthy babies. It stimulates their nervous system and immune system. Well babies who are massaged sleep better through the night, have less colic, and are calmer, as are their mothers. In times of illness, massage, in addition to being comforting, can help relieve your baby's aches, fever, and congestion. Massage can be used to check your baby's body for areas of discomfort or for the small scrapes and bruises that babies get as they learn about their environments. Of course, when serious health problems or injuries occur, consult your pediatrician immediately.

A BLEND OF WEST AND EAST

Infant massage has been common practice among families living in Eastern cultures. For hundreds of years, cultures as diverse as East Indian, African, Jewish, and Japanese have known the benefits of massage and have applied massage to infants. In Asian and African countries, the infant is given a massage with oil following the daily bath before bedtime. Eastern infant massage provides stimulation of internal systems, proper flow of life energy, and relaxation of the muscles. In the Eastern cultures, the tradition of infant massage continues to be passed down from parent to child through the generations.

Although Western countries have been the slowest to use massage in the care of infants, more than ten thousand American mothers currently learn the techniques of infant massage every year. In the United States, the techniques of infant massage are an outgrowth of Swedish massage. Strokes derived from the Western techniques of infant Swedish massage can be used in combination with strokes from Eastern infant massage.

LEARNING HOW TO MASSAGE YOUR BABY

There are specific techniques and massage routines appropriate for infants of different ages and needs. When you blend the techniques and routines with love and nurturance, you and your baby will experience special, intimate times together.

There are systematic approaches to massaging newborns, premature babies, and older infants. Learning how to massage your baby properly will involve a time commitment on your part. It is beyond the scope of this chapter to present a sufficiently detailed description of infant massage for you to apply in a step-by-step fashion. You can read a detailed step-by-step book. You can learn from other parents who are experienced in infant massage. You can watch an educational video. You can take a course and observe others and be shown by experts how to massage your baby. There are institutes all over the United States that teach parents infant massage.

If you have a baby or are expecting a baby, consider learning how to massage your infant. Here are some useful guidelines that will give you an idea of what infant massage is like.

Guidelines for Getting Started

Infant massage begins with a relaxed giver and a relaxed receiver. Relax both your body and mind. Center yourself in preparation for massaging your baby. You can engage in simple breathing exercises and do slow stretches of the tense areas of your body. You can meditate. Relax your shoulders, hands, and wrists. Once you are physically and mentally relaxed, you will be better able to focus on your baby's needs.

Make sure your baby is warm and comfortable. Smile and make eye contact with the baby. Your state of relaxation will communicate safe and pleasant messages, which will help your baby relax and prepare for the massage.

You can give the baby a special cue that it is massage time, for example, by rubbing a small amount of oil into your hands and then showing your oiled palms to the baby. Notice if the baby appears happy and receptive to your touch. Most babies welcome massage. If your baby resists strongly, postpone the massage. Never insist that the baby submit to massage. The child may be ill, cranky, or just not in the mood at that moment. There will be other opportunities for the infant to receive massage.

If the baby is receptive, you can begin the massage by gently removing the baby's clothing. The room should be a comfortable temperature, and your hands should be warm. You should place yourself in a comfortable position that supports you and the baby.

Various seated positions are suggested for the giver during infant massage. During the first weeks or months of the baby's life, holding the baby on your lap will probably work best, since it's a comfortable position for you and a supportive one for the infant. Support your back with a pillow or cushion and sit with your knees slightly bent in the position shown in Figure 6.1.

Guidelines for Massaging Your Baby's Body

Infant massage consists of a variety of strokes, including gentle stretches, rubbing, squeezes, and rolling motions. Some routines begin with the infant's legs and feet and move slowly up the body. Others start with the head and face. As you explore the options, you will find a routine that works best for you and your child. In addition to routines, you can learn and choose from touches and strokes of both Western and Eastern origin. Different types of strokes are recommended for the different parts of the infant's body.

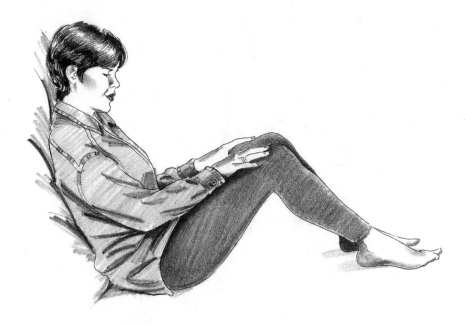

Figure 6.1   A Comfortable Position for Massaging an Infant

The amount of physical pressure you apply in your strokes will vary depending on the baby's age, state of health, and preferences. Over time, you will discover the appropriate amount of pressure to use on different parts of your baby's body if you tune into the feedback your baby gives you. Younger babies and newborns generally require a slower, lighter touch than older infants, but every baby is an individual. Like adults, babies have moods and changing preferences. Your baby might prefer a light touch on some days and a firm touch on others.

Infant massage can effectively blend Eastern and Western techniques so that the baby gets the full benefit of a wide range of nurturing and therapeutic touch practices. We will give you a few examples of infant massage techniques to whet your appetite.

A Flavor of Infant Massage Techniques

You can relax the baby by making gentle circles on the baby's scalp with your fingertips (see Figure 6.2)

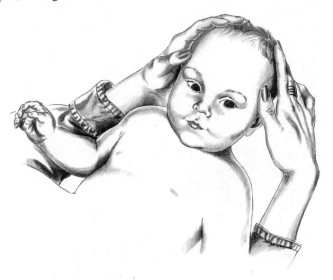

Figure 6.2   Massaging the Infant's Head

Once the baby begins to relax, you can start the actual massage with a rhythmic series of effleurage strokes. These are gentle, but not ticklish, featherlike Swedish strokes that can be applied to the infant's body slowly and evenly from the center to the extremities. Effleurage strokes will help the baby begin to relax and get used to the touch experience.

A technique called *milking*, borrowed from Eastern Indian massage, can be used to relax the baby's arms and legs (see Figures 6.3 and 6.4).

The gentle milking motion pulls tension from the baby's arms and legs. Make sure the baby's skin is lubricated so that your hands glide easily over the baby's arm and leg muscles.

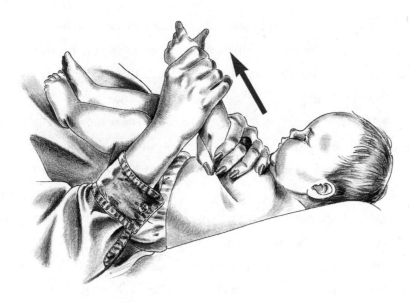

Figure 6.3   "Milking" the Arm, Eastern Style (away from the body)

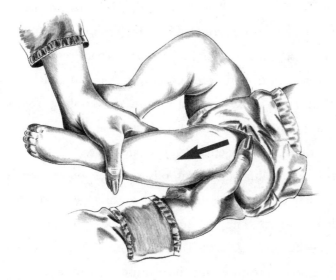

Figure 6.4   "Milking the Leg, Eastern Style (away from the body)

There is a Western format for milking derived from Swedish massage in which the extremity is milked in the direction of the heart, rather than away from the body. The movement of touch toward the heart is intended to promote circulation (see Figure 6.5).

Whether you choose the Eastern or Western version of milking will depend on your goals for the massage and your baby's preference.

If you are short on time, you and your baby can benefit from just a brief foot massage. You can learn to push the sole from heel to toe with your thumbs and squeeze the toes gently, one at a time. Then, push all over the sole with your thumbs to stimulate the nerve endings of the feet (see Figure 6.6).

Massaging the chest begins with light, small, circular motions that soothe the baby and relax the chest muscles. Releasing the tension in the front of the baby's body improves the functioning of the lungs and heart.

Massaging the abdomen can give your baby relief from the discomfort of gas and constipation. When rubbing the abdomen, remember to move your hands clockwise and avoid rubbing the umbilical cord.

Back massage helps strengthen the baby's back muscles and promotes coordinated and flexible movement as your baby approaches increasingly difficult motor tasks, like holding up the head, rolling over, sitting, and eventually crawling, standing, and walking. Like most adults, most babies love the soothing, relaxing effects of back massage.

The Indian and Japanese methods of trigger-point therapy have been adapted for babies. Palpating the baby by pushing gently on the outer layer of muscle can let you know if there are tender spots in the muscles that might be causing pain due to the lack of oxygen and nutrients to those areas. Appropriate finger pressure can relieve muscle spasms and soreness and is a worthwhile adjunct to the techniques adapted from Swedish massage.

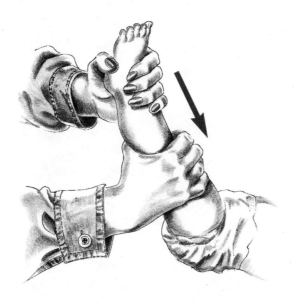

Figure 6.5   "Milking" the Leg, Western Style (toward the heart)

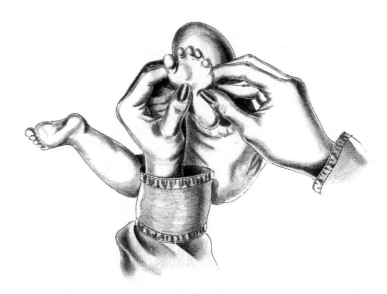

Figure 6.6   Massaging the Infant's Feet

CHAPTER 7

Sports Massage

The purpose of sports massage, also known as performance massage, is to reduce or eliminate factors that interfere with human performance. What sets sports massage apart from other modalities is its emphasis on the prevention of injury.

Sports massage works by loosening and invigorating you both physically and mentally so that you have the best chance of reaching your performance potential. You don't have to be a professional athlete to benefit from sports massage. Any healthy individual engaging in strenuous physical activity is a good candidate for sports massage. If optimum performance, prevention of injury, and restoring yourself when you have completed a strenuous event are among your goals, then sports massage has a place in your life. The sports massage you receive should be tailored to your physical condition and to the nature of your activity.

THE HISTORY AND CURRENT STATUS OF SPORTS MASSAGE

Sports massage originated in Russia in the 1970s. It was developed to help athletes function at maximum capacity by blocking out physical pain during competition. This modality was considered so valuable in the Russian culture that every competing team was assigned a sports massage therapist.

As news of the value of sports massage for optimal physical performance traveled west, research on the effectiveness of this modality was performed in Sweden. In a research study of sports massage in Sweden, competitive cyclists were asked to pedal to the point of exhaustion. Half the cyclists were then given a ten-minute rest, and the other half were given a ten-minute sports massage. After the ten-minute period, all participants did fifty knee extensions. The data revealed that the quadriceps muscles of the massaged cyclists were 11 percent stronger than the quadriceps muscles of the cyclists who rested but received no massage.

It wasn't long before the leaders in American competitive sports heard about the edge provided by sports massage. Johnny Parker, strength coach of the New York Giants, traveled to Russia and learned that providing the players with sports massage could help his team win. The first year that the Giants used sports massage, they won the Super Bowl. Was this a coincidence? Parker didn't think so. He noticed that not only did massage give the team the competitive edge, but it also helped the players heal more quickly from injuries. Receiving sports massage restored their energy and drive.

Another thread in the history and evolution of sports massage in the United States comes from the field of physical therapy. Jack Meagher, a physical therapist, developed the science and art of sports massage in the United States. As a soldier in France during World War II, Meagher received pregame massage (a precursor of today's sports massage) from a German

POW to improve his performance in camp football games. Meagher theorized that muscles that are constantly used become chronically contracted, which makes them less efficient, more exhausted, and more susceptible to injury. Derived from Swedish massage, Meagher's approach to sports massage helps maintain the physical condition of the body, boosts energy and endurance, and promotes ease of movement. Where Meagher's sports massage differs from Swedish is the additional focus on the special needs of athletes to perform at maximum potential, avoid injury, and receive therapeutic touch aimed at restoring mobility to injured areas. Meagher believes that receiving sports massage is so powerful that it can increase performance by 20 percent and actually extend the duration of a professional athlete's career.

The value of sports massage for the health, performance, and vitality of active or athletic individuals is becoming widely recognized. In 1985, the American Massage Therapy Association formed the AMTA National Sports Massage Certification Program, which led to the formation of the AMTA National Sports Massage Team. Certified sports massage therapists are trained not only in the strokes and techniques of massage as applied to athletes but also in anatomy, physiology, and the science of movement.

Since the 1980s, nationally certified sports massage therapists have been on site at the Goodwill, Pan-American, and Olympic games. The 1990s have seen these sports massage therapists routinely at the Boston Marathon, Iron Man competitions, and world-class cycling events.

Many major league teams rely on sports massage for their players before, during, and after games. The Chicago Bulls currently employ six massage therapists for the team, each with individual skills that include relieving muscle spasms, preventing injuries, and alleviating muscle fatigue. The Bulls' strength and conditioning coach, Al Vermeil, implemented this team's massage therapy program in the early 1990s. He believes that sports massage allows athletes to train harder and recover more quickly from exertion and injury.

Major League Baseball teams rely on sports massage to enhance the players' performance. Increasing flexibility, range of motion, and stamina and helping to heal injuries are invaluable benefits for baseball players. Every pitcher for the World Series champion Florida Marlins receives massage throughout each game. All the Marlins receive sports massage for purposes ranging from relieving hamstring injuries to increasing mental focus.

A MODALITY FOR ACTIVE PEOPLE

You do not have to be a professional athlete, a great athlete, or even an athlete at all to benefit from sports massage. It can improve the performance of physically active, healthy individuals who exercise, engage in sports, or have lifestyles and jobs requiring physical strength, agility, and endurance.

Sports massage is intended to loosen and invigorate the individual who engages in any strenuous activity. Such activities may include sports like tennis, racquetball, skiing, soccer, softball, basketball, bicycling, or swimming; exercise in the form of jogging, speed walking, or weight lifting; a major event, like a marathon; or dancing and other performing arts. The activity could even take the form of strenuous physical tasks of daily living, like caring for active children, cooking, and cleaning the house, or a job that requires repeated physical exertion. All of these activities require motivation, the desire to succeed, good coordination and range of motion, physical strength, stamina, and your availability (which means prevention of and quick recovery from injury).

Maximize Your Performance

Sports massage is designed to help you maximize your performance and help you stay active by:

- Enhancing your endurance and stamina.
- Increasing your flexibility and range of motion.
- Preventing you from getting injured.
- Reducing your muscle tension and soreness.
- Increasing the circulation of blood and lymph.
- Enhancing the recovery of your muscles.
- Facilitating the repair of injured soft tissue.
- Relieving your muscle cramps and spasms.

THE STROKES OF SPORTS MASSAGE

When muscle fibers are constricted, blood circulation becomes less efficient. Muscles that are prevented from receiving sufficient oxygen and nutrients carried by the blood through the circulatory system are more susceptible to tension, pain, stiffness, cramps, and spasms. If you enter a strenuous physical event with your muscles in an undernourished condition, you will perform below your potential and be more vulnerable to injury.

Sports massage is designed to spread constricted muscle fibers in order to increase circulation of blood to the muscle tissue. To free the muscle fiber and relieve tension, soreness, stiffness, and pain, the therapist uses a variety of strokes, including:

- Warming the muscles (with a towel, heating pad, or warm hands).
- Direct pressure to the muscles to release painful trigger points.

- ଛ Friction to relieve muscle tension and soreness and to stimulate circulation.
- ଛ Percussion to stimulate and invigorate.
- ଛ Compression (a pumping motion for circulation).
- ଛ Effleurage (gentle, sweeping Swedish strokes).
- ଛ Kneading to help remove waste and toxins.
- ଛ Mild stretching to relieve constriction of muscle fibers and increase range of motion.

These strokes, when applied in the appropriate depth and combination, help prevent injury and aid recuperation. The duration of the massage, depth of touch, and strokes will vary, depending on when the sports massage is given and the condition of the receiver.

THE TIMING OF SPORTS MASSAGE

Sports massage can be received before or after engaging in strenuous activity. When massage is received before the activity, it is called *preevent*. When massage is received after the activity, it is called *postevent*.

Preevent Sports Massage

Preevent sports massage is designed to get your muscles ready for exertion. Although the massage can be full body, the focus will be on those muscles most actively engaged in the upcoming event. For example, if you were facing a bicycle race, the focus would be on your legs, whereas if you were weight lifting, the focus might be on your back and arms. It is important that the most involved muscle groups be in the proper metabolic state in preparation for the event.

Preevent sports massage can be done up to two days before an event. The closer in time to the event, the briefer the massage. The appropriate lengths of sports massage before an event are (1) up to a one-hour massage one to two days prior; (2) a maximum of twenty minutes from ten to twenty-four hours before an event; (3) a ten- to fifteen-minute massage directly preceding or up to ten hours before an event.

Preevent massage can minimize the chances of injury and the impact of injury. Loose, flexible muscles are less prone to injury and muscle spasms than tight, rigid muscles. Preevent massage can also maximize the strength and efficiency of muscles and bodily systems going into an event. Sports massage before an event is meant to be invigorating, not relaxing, in order to stimulate alertness, reaction time, and a positive, winning attitude.

Postevent Sports Massage

During a strenuous physical event, your internal systems, organs, muscles, and brain work overtime. Imagine how hard you have to push yourself to compete successfully against others and against your prior record. Your heart is pumping; you are breathing hard; you are sweating; you are pushing your limits as you do everything you can to motivate yourself to continue to the end. After the event, sports massage can help you eliminate waste products that have accumulated, including lactic acid, and get your body and brain back to a normal, steady state.

Postevent sports massage can be performed immediately following or up to six hours after the event. It is a slower process than preevent massage, since the goal is to return to a normal state rather than to get revved up for action. Postevent sports massage is designed to restore flexibility and muscle tone, reduce muscle tension and soreness, provide relief from muscle

Benefits of Sports Massage

BEFORE AN EVENT:

Optimal performance.

Enhanced endurance and stamina.

More flexibility and range of motion.

Injury prevention.

Less muscle tension and soreness.

Increased circulation of blood and lymph.

Invigorated bodily systems and brain.

Enhanced alertness and mental focus.

AFTER AN EVENT:

Faster recovery of your muscles.

Faster removal of lactic acid.

Faster repair of soft tissue.

Increased circulation of blood and lymph.

Relief from muscle cramps and spasms.

Revival of sore and tired muscle tissue.

Return to homeostasis.

spasms and cramps, and reduce the immediate and long-term impact of injury to muscle tissue. After a strenuous event, you can suffer subtle damage to the microfibers of your muscle tissue. Sports massage helps restore and repair damage to soft tissue by increasing the circulation of blood and lymph. The oxygen and other nutrients supplied by the blood, in combination with the lymphatic elimination of waste and toxins from the muscle tissue, facilitate muscle repair. The better the condition of your muscles, the faster you can return to training.

Sports massage can enhance your safety and enjoyment when vigorous activity is a part of your life. This modality is considered so effective that it can actually extend the working life of a career athlete.

ENHANCED PERFORMANCE FOR MARATHON RUNNERS

Robert Blasi, a licensed massage therapist in New Jersey, provided sports massage to runners preparing for the 1998 New York City Marathon. These runners considered sports massage an essential component of their training program.

In his work with runners, Blasi focused on their lower body, legs, and pained areas. One client had such extreme pain in his shins that he thought he would not be able to participate in the marathon. Blasi used an eclectic approach that combined Swedish massage, neuromuscular therapy, and myofascial release. He also incorporated stretching into the sports massage. This client got off Blasi's table feeling he could run the marathon right then and there.

ENHANCED PERFORMANCE FOR SWIMMERS

Blasi, along with Andrew Levine, provided sports massage to the Rutgers University Women's Swimming Team. The head coach, Chuck Warner, believes that providing therapeutic massage to his athletes aids in post-training recovery. About 90 percent of the bodywork given to the swimmers focused on the rotator cuff. The head coach stated that these massage therapists were "highly effective in accelerating recovery time for our athletes."

The Rutgers swimmers expressed gratitude to the massage therapists for alleviating the tension in their muscles and for relief from the chronic pain that can accompany overtraining. The swimmers also felt that the sports massage helped increase their stamina and endurance, making them more competitive.

CHAPTER 8

Geriatric Massage

The term *geriatric* refers to the process of aging. Geriatric massage, a modality derived from Swedish massage, is designed for the special needs of older adults. The physical, social, and psychological consequences of aging have been taken into account in the development of geriatric massage.

One goal of massage for older adults is to provide nurturing touch to individuals who, because of the life circumstances that accompany aging, may be suffering from touch deprivation. Stress, anxiety, and depression can increase over time, which will have an adverse impact on physical health. Another goal of massage for older adults is to increase and maintain flexibility of movement and improve blood circulation, both of which need extra attention as we age.

In some ways, geriatric massage is similar to sports or performance massage. Like the athlete who receives massage to perform at a peak level, geriatric massage can aid the geriatric population to function at optimal capacity. The strokes are designed to increase range of motion and improve mobility. However, the geriatric population has limitations that do not apply to the athletic population. Unlike athletes, most older adults must be touched with special gentleness, and many have health problems that should be considered by the massage therapist.

WHO IS INCLUDED IN THE GERIATRIC POPULATION?

Age seventy-five has been pinpointed as the starting point in the population termed *geriatric*. The geriatric population is the fastest-growing population in North America. The continual development and refinement of medication and medical procedures that support and even take over body systems and functions are enabling people to live much longer. Because an increasing life span is a relatively new issue in society, we are learning the ramifications of living past the seventies, eighties, and even nineties.

The new advances in medicine have enhanced the quality of life for many elderly adults. For those fortunate enough to maintain relatively good health and coping skills, living longer has provided the opportunity to continue exploring their interests and enjoying their relationships.

Unfortunately, there are those for whom life is longer but unsatisfying. Not all members of the geriatric population feel well or cope well with the many profound changes that accompany aging. Health problems, financial problems, loss of independence, loneliness, and fear of death are among the issues that trouble many people over age seventy-five. In general, those who have resolved crises at earlier stages of development in a rational, productive way will cope more effectively with aging than those who have been prone to anxiety and depression all along the journey.

Aging and Health

The geriatric population suffers from health problems due to the physiological wear and tear of the aging process. No one who lives a long life completely escapes the ravages of aging. Many individuals over the age of seventy-five demonstrate declines in metabolism, body fluid, kidney filtration rate, cardiac output, oxygen uptake, breathing rate, nerve impulse travel, reaction time, strength of grip, blood flow to the brain, and even brain weight. These declines create other problems. For example, the reduction of cardiac output results in increased blood pressure, which can lead to vascular constriction and disease. The reduction in blood circulation can lead to loss of elasticity of the muscle and connective tissue, restricted joint movement, and numbness in the extremities. These conditions contribute to poor mobility, unsteadiness of gait, osteoporosis, and falling, which can result in fractures and breaks in brittle bones.

The physical decline is accompanied by social and emotional issues. Major challenges for the elderly include coping with loss, fear of more loss, and frustration over increasing dependency. The loss through death of friends, spouse, and other family members triggers feelings of loneliness, fear, and sadness. Perhaps the most difficult losses involve the losses in oneself. Coping with the multiple losses of youth, strength, attractiveness, good health, sharp skills, freedom of movement, and energy can feel overwhelming. Because of these changes and the knowledge that the losses will only increase, depression is not unusual among the elderly.

The nurturing and therapeutic powers of touch can provide a feeling of connection, improved health, and hope. Unfortunately, for many older adults, touch becomes more infrequent. As their health declines and the losses mount, there are fewer people in their world to touch them. Except for doing standard medical procedures, many nurses avoid touching the elderly who are acutely ill. The lack of touch adds to the already profound feelings of isolation and depression. Lack of tactile stimulation can also contribute to the sluggishness of the body's internal systems. Geriatric massage provides the kind of touch and stimulation that is designed to promote the physical and mental health of older adults.

Variations in Health Status

For some people, the emotional and mental problems and losses that accompany aging have devastating effects. Other individuals are more adaptable. You can think of the geriatric population as loosely divided into three groups:

1. Robust individuals who are healthy, active, and feel young for their age.
2. Age-appropriate individuals (the largest group) who are active but have some health problems and need special care during massage.
3. Frail individuals who have serious health problems and need the gentlest treatment of all.

The geriatric massage therapist takes a careful history to determine the health status of each client. The approach to massage varies with the needs of each individual.

DIETRICH MIESLER AND
THE GERIATRIC MASSAGE PROJECT

Dietrich Miesler learned about massage as a young man in Germany in the 1940s, but it was not until the 1970s that he began to focus on it as a career. After studying massage in San Francisco, he worked as a massage therapist in a nursing home. He combined work with education and earned his bachelor's degree from San Jose State University, where he majored in German and psychology. Miesler earned a master's degree in health science and a certificate in gerontology.

Through his education and hands-on experience massaging the geriatric population in nursing home environments, Miesler acquired a vast knowledge of the application of massage to older adults. He became a nursing home administrator, but his real dream was to develop a massage modality geared to the needs of the geriatric population and to teach massage therapists how to work effectively with aging adults.

To realize this dream, Miesler founded the Geriatric Massage Project in Sebastopol, California, in 1991 when he was sixty-six. It was the first project of its kind in the United States to focus on the special touch needs of the elderly. The purpose of the Geriatric Massage Project is to gather and disseminate information about this population from a variety of fields, including medicine, sociology, psychology, and bodywork.

Massage is viewed as a healthy, nurturing treatment for the many physical and emotional problems that accompany aging. The techniques developed by Miesler and his program are practical and targeted at providing comforting touch and promoting health in this growing population.

The educational programs and materials developed and disseminated by the Geriatric Massage Project have so far trained more than one thousand massage therapists all over the country in the specialty of geriatric massage. The newsletter distributed by the Geriatric Massage Project contains information on formal training programs, videotapes, readings, equipment (e.g., special bolsters that suit the limbs of the elderly), and health issues relevant to treating this population.

EXPERIENCING GERIATRIC MASSAGE

Geriatric massage is a rewarding experience for both the receiver and the giver. The compassion and warmth communicated through geriatric massage create a special connection between therapist and client. In a successful geriatric massage, the therapist is in tune with the client as a unique human being with special needs.

For the purposes of this book, the experience of geriatric massage will focus on the robust and age-appropriate categories rather than the frail. Geriatric massage begins with an assessment of the client's health.

Assessment

A thorough health history is taken in order to determine the most beneficial approach to the massage and whether there are any contraindications. The massage will be tailored to the client's needs, taking into account information from the health history that indicates the need to avoid touching certain parts of the body or to treat certain areas with extra care.

Sometimes, the massage therapist will ask your permission to consult your physician before scheduling the massage. In addition, you, as the client, might want to consult your physician if you are considering massage. If you suffer from heart disease, high blood pressure, peripheral vascular disease, thrombosis, diabetes, or constipation, a doctor's permission is needed to perform geriatric massage. Sharing your health conditions with the massage therapist and allowing the therapist to consult with your physician will ensure that you receive a safe, beneficial massage.

Getting Started

As in Swedish massage, the geriatric client is draped with a towel or sheet on a padded massage table. Modesty is respected at all times, just as it is with clients of all ages.

Most geriatric massage will last a maximum of thirty minutes. A full-hour massage might be too much stimulation of the nervous and circulatory systems for this age group. The desired level of stimulation of internal systems during massage for the geriatric population is below that of younger individuals.

Like Swedish massage, geriatric massage is a full-body massage, except for those areas that might be contraindicated or any areas that the receiver does not want touched. The massage begins with gentle rocking motions, calming strokes, and some deep breaths for relaxation. Once the receiver is relaxed and accustomed to the situation, the massage therapist will apply the strokes of geriatric massage.

The Strokes of Geriatric Massage

The strokes of geriatric massage are light and gentle hand motions. The pressure is always comfortable and soothing to the muscles. Nothing is ever forced. Medical considerations are always taken into account in order to adjust the strokes and depth of touch to the needs of each individual.

Gentle rocking and shaking motions are used to lull the body into a state of relaxation. These subtle movements signal the nervous system to release endorphins that produce pleasurable sensations. The interplay between body and mind can have a welcome relaxing effect on the receiver.

Most of the massage consists of Swedish effleurage strokes, as well as adaptations of effleurage designed to meet the needs of this special population. The effleurage strokes are a gentle succession of featherlike movements done with the tips of the therapist's fingers. These strokes provide light stimulation of the nerve endings. When applied in a slow, rhythmic fashion, effleurage strokes produce feelings of warmth, comfort, and relaxation. The massage strokes are applied in the direction of the flow of blood and lymph, to stimulate the circulation of these vital fluids. Effleurage can help reduce feelings of restlessness, reduce headaches, and promote better sleep.

Miesler created what are known as hybrid strokes, or strokes that are a combination of more than one stroke. One such stroke, known as fluffing, combines effleurage with petrissage, another Swedish massage stroke. Fluffing is a gentle, repetitive, and therapeutic massage stroke specifically developed by Miesler for the geriatric population. The goal of fluffing is to boost circulation in, or "fluff up," the muscles. The increased circulation encourages the rebuilding of muscle fiber, which can become protein-deficient during the aging process.

Although the techniques are light and gentle, the impact of geriatric massage can be profound. Using fluffing and other hybrid strokes, Miesler once saved a client's legs that had been scheduled for amputation.

BENEFITS OF GERIATRIC MASSAGE

The benefits of geriatric massage are all interconnected. Each health benefit has a ripple effect throughout the body's systems. The physical and mental health benefits are interrelated as well. Feeling better physically, feeling less pain, and moving more freely lift the spirits. Feeling less depressed and more optimistic improves the ability to cope with health problems. Keep these connections in mind as you read the specific benefits.

Geriatric massage increases circulation. The circulatory system consists of blood and lymph vessels. It is responsible for the distribution of oxygen, for nourishment, and for hormonal releases from the endocrine system. The circulation of lymph removes carbon monoxide and the waste products of cell repair and replacement. Miesler regards the positive impact of geriatric massage on the circulation of blood and lymph as the greatest benefit of this modality, because almost all individuals in this population suffer a decline in the efficiency and health of their circulatory systems.

Geriatric massage stimulates the nervous system. Miesler believes that the stiffness of the muscles in the elderly is due not only to localized problems but also to a breakdown in communication between the mind and the body. It is the open flow of communication from brain to body and body to brain that keeps the body flexible. Once this communication breaks down, muscles can stay tense even when the individual does not feel mentally stressed, because the nervous system fails to release the chemicals that allow the muscles to relax. The touch of geriatric massage is designed to reestablish the mind-body connection via stimulation of the nervous system through the power of touch.

Geriatric massage softens muscle tissue and connective tissue that have hardened over the years. The strokes of geriatric massage relieve muscle tension and pain by increasing the flow of oxygen and other nutrients to the affected areas. As the muscles relax and the connective tissue surrounding them softens, range of motion, gait disorders, and mobility can improve. Some specific movement-related problems that respond to geriatric massage include fractures, joint replacements, stroke-induced paralysis, joint stiffness, and nervous movement disorders, including Parkinson's disease.

Nurses and family members have noticed that the need for pain medication is often reduced when the geriatric patient undergoes massage. The medical condition may persist, but the symptoms are relieved along with the individual's level of stress about the condition. The reduction of mental tension that results from geriatric massage has a positive impact on both physical and mental health. The receiver feels energized and more alive.

Geriatric massage decreases mental tension through the release of endorphins, the brain's natural opiates. Mental relaxation triggers overall feelings of well-being and inner peace. The lowered mental tension, tranquilizing effect, and improved bodily functions promoted by geriatric massage help this population with insomnia, which is maintained by a number of physical conditions and by emotional distress. The improved digestion and elimination provided by massage can trigger a better appetite and emotional outlook.

Geriatric massage helps fight depression. The inevitable changes and losses that accompany aging trigger negative thinking, fear, and bouts of depression in this population. The compassionate touch of massage counteracts the chemistry that maintains depression and makes the receiver feel connected, nurtured, worthwhile, and cared for. These feelings enhance the quality of life.

The givers of geriatric massage benefit as well. Providing this level of nurturing, hands-on care can increase the giver's sensitivity and appreciation of the value of compassionate giving. Being in tune with the geriatric receiver makes the giver confront his or her vulnerability and mortality, insights that can lead to a richer life.

Benefits of Geriatric Massage

Improved circulation of blood and lymph.

Improved digestion, appetite, and elimination.

Cells receive more oxygen and other nutrients.

Stimulation of the nervous system.

Reduced muscle tension and pain.

Improved mobility and gait.

Reduction in movement symptoms of Parkinson's disease.

Better communication between mind and body.

Improved mental relaxation.

Improved quality of sleep.

The providing of nurturing touch.

Relief from depression.

CHAPTER 9

Myofascial Release Therapy

Myofascial release, also known as myofascial massage therapy and deep-tissue massage, is a deeper Western massage modality than Swedish. It is a powerful modality focused on lasting pain relief. Whereas Swedish massage addresses only the muscles, myofascial release addresses the fascia, the tissue that surrounds and connects the muscles, bones, and internal organs. *Myo* means "muscle." *Myofascial* refers to both muscle and fascia. Myofascial release treats the whole body and is aimed at releasing tension in the fascia as a means of restoring balance to the body and its systems.

JOHN F. BARNES AND MYOFASCIAL RELEASE THERAPY

John F. Barnes is a physical therapist who is known as a pioneer in the study of fascia and its application to myofascial release therapy. Barnes considers fascia the missing link in traditional medical approaches to pain management. He believes that chronic pain cannot be alleviated long-term without treating the fascia, the pervasive three-dimensional weblike substance that runs throughout the entire internal structure of the body. Barnes has developed an eclectic approach that combines myofascial release therapy with craniosacral therapy.

Unfortunately, most traditional doctors become overly focused on the symptom—the pain—rather than on its underlying cause. Since they ignore the existence of the fascial system, they do not address the problems there that maintain chronic pain. As a result, many patients can only get temporary symptom relief, usually through medication, because the snags, restrictions, and distortions in the fascia remain uncorrected.

Barnes considers this deficiency in the medical model a serious one that makes this aspect of traditional medicine antiquated. Barnes believes that myofascial assessment and therapy should be incorporated into the medical care of pain syndromes because its biochemical, bioelectrical, and neurophysiological effects help relieve pain from its source. By including the fascial system in the assessment and treatment of pain, practitioners of this modality, whether medically trained or not, can eliminate the cause of pain systematically and with long-lasting results.

FUN FACTS ABOUT FASCIA

Understanding the mechanisms and benefits of myofascial release therapy begins with knowledge about fascia and the fascial system. You can think of the fascia as resembling plastic wrap but with the consistency of the filmy, slippery tissue surrounding a skinless chicken breast. This connective tissue provides the body with strength, support, elasticity, and cushion. It protects

the organs and provides contour to
the limbs. Fascia also provides a covering that helps conserve body heat
(see Figure 9.1).

By releasing the fascia from
clinging too tightly and rigidly to muscle tissue, myofascial release therapy
can provide a deep release of long-
standing physical pain and mental
tension. Following are some fun and
informative facts about fascia.

It Is Everywhere

Fascia is found everywhere in the
body. It wraps around and through
the muscles, giving them shape and
support. Fascia encases all the organs,
veins, and arteries. It comes together
at the ends of muscles to form tendons, which attach to the bones.

Fascia covers every muscle, every
muscle fiber, and every muscle fibril
(the smallest unit of the muscle) and
even extends to the cellular level. It

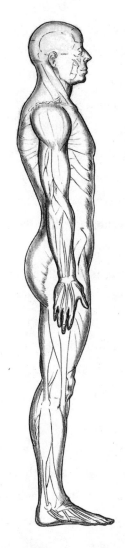

Figure 9.1   Fascia Throughout the Body

surrounds every cell in the body where the interstitial fluids are held. These
fluids contain platelets, lymph, and other life-supporting substances.
Because fascia plays a major role in the circulation of vital fluids, and

because it surrounds everything so completely that it gives your body shape, it is important to maintain its health.

You Can Squeeze It

Fascia, when healthy, is well hydrated and holds water in its ground substance at the cellular level. Healthy fascia is pliable and moves freely with the locomotion of the body. Pliability means that it has give. Hydration of the fascia allows for a healthy interchange of nutrients and waste products.

When not healthy and hydrated, due to stress or injury, fascia can become rigid, fibrotic, and glued down. Impaired movement and degenerative processes will result.

Fascia is not easily squeezable in this state. It can become hard as a rock as it sticks fast to the cells, muscles, bones, and organs it surrounds. Just imagine what happens inside of you when your fascia hardens, crowding your muscles, cells, and organs and no longer acting as a comfortable, pliable cushion.

It Cushions, Shapes, Separates, and Supports

Fascia is a substance that *cushions* us from external assault, gives our bodies *shape* and contour, *separates* our muscles, even our cells, from each other, and *supports* our muscles, bones, and internal organs.

One of the main functions of fascia is to act as a shock absorber. Healthy fascia takes in energy and acts as a cushion. Its ability to change from a solid to a gellike consistency is what makes it cushiony.

Fascia gets its qualities from the substances it comprises.

1. *Collagen,* a protein that ensures there are no weak points and provides strength to guard against overextension.

2. *Elastin,* another protein substance, which is rubberlike and absorbs movement. Elastin contains parallel fibers that are laid down in areas where elasticity is required, as in the skin and arteries.

3. *Polysaccharide gel complex,* a gelatinous substance that fills the spaces between the fibers. This gel complex serves several important functions. For one, it forms the gel of the ground substance, which absorbs compressive forces of movement. It also lubricates the collagen, elastin, and muscle fibers so that they can move over each other with minimal friction.

Fascia protects your organs by dispersing subtle impacts to your physical structure. This process prevents any one area from being overstressed.

Its plastic nature enables healthy fascia to adapt appropriately to movements and changes in the body. In fact, fascia is involved in all aspects of motion. As long as forces are not too great, the gel of the ground substance can absorb the shock of sudden movements or compressive forces, dispersing the impact throughout the body.

Thus, fascia is a support system for the body's inherent tendency to right itself. It supports and facilitates the contraction and movements of muscles and supports the bones in a dynamic balance with the soft tissue, giving you structure and support.

If fascia is restricted at the time of trauma, or the force is too great, the impact cannot be dispersed properly, and isolated areas will be overstressed. A person whose fascia does not have enough give can suffer severe injury.

It's All Connected

In addition to being everywhere and covering everything, large and small, throughout the body, and in addition to being gelatinous, pliable, three-dimensional, and strong, fascia is also entirely interconnected. It is like one huge, winding, squeezable web of taffy. It is because of its being interconnected that gluing or sticking of the fascia to any one area will affect other parts of the body. Fascia acts like a thick knit sweater that resides between your skin and your bones (see Figure 9.2). One pull in the knit may affect the weave in both surrounding and distant areas. This pull may cause torquing of the underlying structure, resulting in pain patterns that are remote from the original site.

Abnormal Fascia—Not So Much Fun

If your fascia enters an abnormal state, you can develop poor posture or even structural misalignments. Fascia in poor condition can erode, calcify, or crystallize. It can displace bones out of their proper placement. Blood vessels and nerves could be encroached upon.

Abnormal fascia may cause widespread toxicity and pain. When the systems of the body are suffocating because the fascia has tightened around them, the soft tissue becomes deprived of water, oxygen, and nutrients, deficiencies that lead to a condition known as ischemia. Ischemia makes the areas deprived of oxygen feel painful to the touch.

Abnormal fascia may cause loss of flexibility, gait disturbances, organ displacement, and even energy-draining postures that wear you down, causing fatigue and depression. In essence, abnormal fascia can speed up the aging process. Even worse—or maybe just as bad, depending on your point of view—the problems caused by untreated, abnormal fascia include emo-

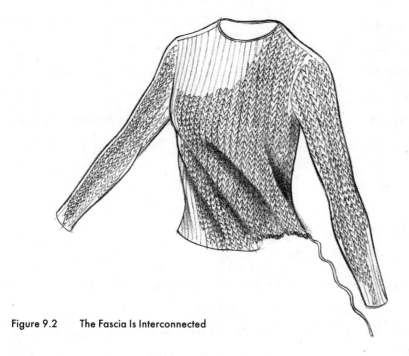

Figure 9.2   The Fascia Is Interconnected

tional armoring and self-protective holding patterns that are associated with dependency, depression, and disability.

EXPERIENCING THE EMPOWERMENT
OF MYOFASCIAL RELEASE

Rather than taking a passive stance (as you would in Swedish and manual lymph drainage), you, as the client, are an active participant in myofascial massage therapy. The client and the massage therapist plan the course of treatment together in a collaborative fashion. The client remains active during treatment by providing ongoing feedback to the massage therapist regarding location of pain and desired intensity and duration of the therapeutic touch.

Your active role in the process of myofascial massage can enhance not only the release of physical pain and tension but also feelings of empowerment with regard to your health and well-being. The feelings of empowerment that you produce by perceiving yourself as a participant in your own healing process, rather than as a victim of your physical and emotional pain, go a long way in helping you overcome self-denigrating thought patterns and negative emotions.

ASSESSMENT AND TREATMENT IN MYOFASCIAL RELEASE

Myofascial release is a whole-body approach that helps the various parts of the body work together in harmony. When a part of the body is injured, mistreated, overutilized, or neglected, it becomes divorced from the rest of the body. Myofascial release provides a mechanism through which these malfunctioning, rejected parts are welcomed back to the rest of the body. The massage therapist, through gentle, persistent strokes aimed at coaxing the fascia to release, signals the body to integrate its separate parts into a whole, functioning system. The reintegration of the body is an important focus in the process of myofascial release.

The Assessment Phase

In order for the client and therapist to achieve the goals that this powerful modality offers, they must agree on the purpose of the work, come to a common understanding of the possible outcomes, and make a commitment to the therapy. Your commitment is important because whatever your fascial abnormalities may be, they did not develop overnight. They are too deeply entrenched to be corrected in just one session.

It is not uncommon for clients not to feel profound effects until at least twenty-four hours following a treatment. Committing to three sessions will let you know if the modality is working for you. To quote Hippocrates, "Healing takes time." This modality requires patience on the part of both therapist and client.

Because myofascial release is a whole-body approach, it would not be uncommon for a myofascial therapist to do a postural analysis of a client. The purpose of doing a postural analysis is to uncover bodily distortions such as rounded shoulders, anterior pelvic tilt (pelvis tipped to the front of the body), pronation of the feet, collapsed arches, and protracted head syndrome.

For the fascia to remain optimally functional, bodily distortions need to be noted during assessment and then addressed during treatment. Take the pelvis, a central focus of this modality. When the pelvis tips to one side or the other and turns away from its horizontal position in relation to gravity, the body becomes more prone to postural distortions because gravity will pull it down. Think about the positioning of your head in relation to the rest of your body. For every inch that the head's center of gravity is shifted abnormally forward, the lower back is subjected to a force equivalent to the additional weight of your head. The average head weighs 12 pounds. According to this formula, if your head goes three inches forward, that's 36 pounds of extra pressure on the lower back. These distortions create adaptive compensations, which, in turn, cause snagging and torquing of the fascia.

A snag in one area of the fascia has the potential of distorting other areas of fascia, which can be located far from the obvious area of trauma. Because the fascia is intertwined around the muscles, veins, and arteries, a pull in one location can create problems in distant areas. This is why the myofascial therapist treats the body as a whole, even if the client comes in with a specific complaint.

As part of the assessment process, a hands-on evaluation through pal-pation of the soft tissue may aid the massage therapist in creating a treat-ment plan. The therapist's experience and intuition help him or her locate painful areas and holding patterns, which will direct the course of treatment.

A thorough assessment also includes a knowledge of the history of the client's body, including physical traumas that occurred in the past. Boundary issues are also discussed in the beginning to help establish trust between giver and receiver. Establishing appropriate boundaries is an important part of the foundation of treatment.

The Treatment Phase

The myofascial release therapist begins with the treatment plan formed dur-ing the assessment phase, based on the information obtained by talking with and examining the client. This plan may be modified as treatment pro-gresses and new feedback is obtained as the therapist works on your body.

Myofascial release can be done with the client in loose, comfortable clothing, partially clothed, in just underwear, or unclothed, depending on the client's preference. Oil is not used, because the myofascial therapist has to be able to feel the release in the muscle or fascia. Oil might make the sur-face of the skin too slippery. Friction is desirable because it aids the release. Myofascial therapy is done slowly and patiently. It is directional, done on certain angles determined by the structure of the tissue.

To help the client adapt to treatment and feel comfortable with it, the first contacts are very gentle. The muscles and superficial layer of fascia are warmed so that they become loosened up and more receptive to deeper touch. The progression in myofascial release is from superficial to deep. As the session progresses, the therapist will be constantly monitoring for myofascial releases and remain in communication with the client regarding moving ahead in the treatment.

The strokes used in myofascial release are designed to bring back the original consistency of the substances that make up the fascia. One stroke used in myofascial release is called skin rolling, a movement in which the therapist lifts the skin away from the bone while bunching and creeping the fingers across the area. Skin rolling is a helpful technique because it can alert the therapist to holding patterns deep in the affected areas.

The therapist uses prolonged light pressure in the direction of fascial restriction to allow the tissues to release. Strokes called compression (both static and twisting) may be used by the therapist in thicker areas of fascia.

In addition to using massage strokes designed to gently release the fascia, the therapist also assesses and treats craniosacral rhythms. Adding this dimension to the fascial treatment helps make the positive results last longer. (For information on the craniosacral system and craniosacral therapy, please refer to chapter 15 of this book.)

Having identified areas of restricted movement, the therapist will determine the best course of action. Techniques to unblock the restriction include softening, lengthening, lifting, broadening, and separating the fascia. At appropriate points in treatment, the therapist may ask the client to play an active role by moving a body part while another area is pinned by the therapist. This type of movement facilitates the stretching of the fascia. As treatment progresses and the client becomes increasingly tolerant of deeper work, the therapist moves from superficial to deep, using the thumbs, fingertips, and forearms to sink into the soft tissue and release the fascia.

The therapist needs both patience and sensitivity to coax the fascia into release and to feel the release. As the client, you are instructed by the therapist to utilize breathing techniques designed to aid the release process. Breathing up into the affected area may expedite the softening of the tissue. By working as an active member of the partnership with the therapist to release the fascia, the client feels empowered.

Enmeshed with the physical tension of tight and hardened fascia are also long-held emotions that became trapped in our bodies through the stress and distortions they caused. It would not be unusual during myofascial release to release some feelings as well. If you want to say something verbally that contains emotional content, the massage therapist will not be surprised. This is not to say that myofascial release is a form of psychotherapy. It is not. However, the receiver's experience and expression of emotion are legitimate parts of the process.

WHEN IS TREATMENT COMPLETED?

Treatment is completed when fascial restrictions are removed and the body's equilibrium has been restored. You will know that this has happened. Your body will return to a balanced state and become realigned with the force of gravity. Your body will function freer from restrictions. Your body's natural ability to self-correct will be restored. You will be able to expend your energy in a more efficient way, free of pain.

Between sessions and at the end of treatment, the myofascial massage therapist will suggest certain stretching exercises intended to help you maintain the gains made in treatment.

BENEFITS OF MYOFASCIAL RELEASE

Many people opt for myofascial release to alleviate chronic pain, tension, poor range of motion, and poor posture. This modality is known for relieving muscle tightness in the neck, jaw, and back, and for relieving the pain of acute injuries, such as those due to sports. In addition to alleviating pain, releasing the fascia gives the organs room in which to function. Strain is reduced and respiration improves. Myofascial release has successfully treated scoliosis.

As myofascial imbalances are restored, body awareness increases, movement becomes relaxed and natural, and your physical structure will become more aligned with gravity. This will improve your posture and help maintain the gains obtained through the myofascial release process.

Participating in this massage modality can create positive changes on an even deeper level. When you become free of long-standing pain, including chronic discomfort that lingers in the background and interferes subtly with the quality of your sleep, you can become mentally and emotionally drained. As you allow the fascia to be released, you also may shed some of the mental tension and emotional distress that has built up over time and has become encased in the rigidified fascia. This type of release can free your mental energy and emotional spontaneity.

WHEN TO AVOID OR POSTPONE MYOFASCIAL RELEASE

If you suffer from any of the following conditions, you should not undergo myofascial release treatments: malignancies, aneurysm, acute rheumatoid arthritis. Areas of your body that contain open wounds, serious bruises, or fractures should not be exposed to myofascial release. Be sure to be open and accurate during the assessment phase of the myofascial release process so that the therapist has the opportunity to determine if you are an appropriate candidate for the treatment.

Benefits of Myofascial Release

Relief from chronic pain and physical tension.

Increased range of motion.

Relief from muscle tightness in many areas, including the neck, jaw, and back.

Relief from the pain of acute injuries, including sports injuries.

Relief from scoliosis.

Organs have more room in which to function.

Improved respiration.

Increased body awareness.

More relaxed and natural movement.

Alignment of your physical structure with gravity.

Improved posture.

Enhanced mental clarity and emotional spontaneity.

TRAINING IN MYOFASCIAL RELEASE

There is no one formal institution where a massage therapist can become trained and certified as a myofascial release practitioner. Many massage therapists are introduced to the theory and practice of myofascial release during their training as massage therapists. After that, specialization takes the form of workshops, seminars, and continuing education, offered by the MFR Treatment Center and Seminars established by John Barnes.

More than twenty thousand practitioners have been trained through these seminars. The types of professionals who undertake specialized training in myofascial release include massage therapists, physical therapists, and medical doctors.

MYOFASCIAL RELEASE
HAS CHANGED PEOPLE'S LIVES

The improvement in emotional state and outlook that accompanies the relief from chronic pain makes myofascial release therapy a powerful force in the lives of many of those who experience it. Cheryl Mulligan, a myofascial release therapist in New Jersey, receives letters from her grateful clients telling her, "You've changed my life."

One of her clients, an executive in his thirties, suffered for years from bulging discs and extreme tightness in his lower back. He found no relief until he tried myofascial release therapy. He experienced immediate alleviation after the first half hour of treatment. Cheryl explained, "He felt instant relief. The doctor had talked with him about surgery, but he doesn't want to have the surgery. I think he's going to keep up with the massage, and we'll keep an eye on it."

Another client, Jean Scarpa, was diagnosed with fibromyalgia in April 1996 and was taking medication to make it through the day. She began receiving myofascial release therapy twice a week from Cheryl in May 1997. By July 1997, she no longer used drugs for pain relief and saw Cheryl and a chiropractor once a week.

Jean wrote in a letter about her experience: "I truly feel that the combination of both of these techniques [chiropractic and myofascial release] helped me to get off the drugs. These treatments have let me know that I can still lead a fulfilling life that is free from the drugs whose only purpose was to mask the consistent, chronic pain. . . . I do not know where I would be without the benefits of massage therapy. Please spread the word so that people who suffer as I do may try this alternative to drugs."

Releasing Points of Stress

Neuromuscular Therapy

Shiatsu

Reflexology

The modalities covered in this section focus on relieving pain, improving health, and enhancing the mind-body connection by releasing specific points of stress. Whereas neuromuscular therapy is a Western modality, shiatsu and reflexology are Eastern in origin. Differences in Western and Eastern philosophies and approaches to healing are brought to light in this section of the book.

CHAPTER 10

Neuromuscular Therapy

Neuromuscular therapy, or NMT, is a scientific bodywork modality designed to relieve trigger points and chronic muscular pain syndromes. The process of neuromuscular therapy is precise and requires NMT practitioners to have specialized knowledge of neuromuscular anatomy and intensive training in its application to alleviating muscular pain.

When you are free of pain, the systems and structures of your body work together in harmony. However, when you are in pain, the functioning of your body is off, or out of balance. This imbalance occurs partly because of our natural tendency to compensate for the pain in one area of the body by overusing and thereby creating stress on other muscles that are not in pain.

A major goal of NMT is to locate the sources of pain, free you of the pain, and help restore and maintain the proper balance of the body, bringing it back into harmony. This state of harmony or balance is known as homeostasis. NMT renews structural homeostasis by restoring normal physiological functioning between the central nervous system (the brain, spinal cord, and nerves) and the musculoskeletal system (the skeleton and muscles of the body).

The process of freeing the body of chronic pain and restoring homeostasis is accomplished in NMT by locating and treating trigger points: tender, sensitive areas in the soft tissue that (1) are painful to the touch, and (2) refer or send pain to other parts of the body, which can be far removed from the trigger point itself. The successful treatment of trigger points can bring lasting relief from long-standing chronic pain syndromes.

DR. JANET TRAVELL AND
THE SIGNIFICANCE OF TRIGGER POINTS

The focus of the neuromuscular therapy bodywork modality is on the relief of pain and pain syndromes occurring from trigger points—small, hypersensitive knots or ropelike bands that can be found in body tissue, including the muscles, the fascia, the cutaneous section of the skin, ligaments, the tissue surrounding the bone, and even in scars. Trigger points usually occur at the junction of the nerve and the muscle in areas that are lacking in oxygen.

The term *trigger point* was coined by Janet G. Travell, M.D., whose life work was the study and application of the impact of the body's chemistry on muscle pain. She discovered the existence and importance of trigger points when she worked with patients as a physician at New York Hospital, Cornell Medical College Center, on the pulmonary, cardiology, and general medical service units. Her careful observations of her patients' pain complaints led her to investigate trigger points and how they function.

From the 1950s until her death in 1997, Travell created the science of trigger-point therapy, a field of medicine that did not exist before. NMT is considered a form of trigger-point therapy. During those four decades, Travell was a researcher, teacher, and practitioner who filled a significant void in the area of pain management. She provided care for Senator John F. Kennedy five years before his election as president and became the first woman to serve as a physician to an American president. She continued as White House physician through the Johnson administration. Travell and those practitioners trained in her techniques have been able to relieve chronic pain for individuals who have not obtained relief elsewhere.

Most individuals who undergo NMT have tried something else first, including home remedies, consulting either their family doctor, a medical specialist, or a chiropractor, and have not obtained sufficient or long-lasting relief. In the case of medical treatment, part of the reason for the lack of chronic pain resolution is that most medical doctors do not examine soft tissue manually and therefore do not locate trigger points. Rather, they listen to the patient's complaint, rule out clear-cut life-threatening medical bases for the pain, like cancer or heart disease (which is an important diagnostic step), and then prescribe pain medication. Unfortunately, pain medication works imperfectly. It wears off, can have side effects almost as unpleasant as the original pain symptom, and can lead to drug tolerance and increasing dosages.

Chiropractors address the pain more directly than medical doctors, but their domain is limited to bone structure and bone adjustment. Chiropractors do not manipulate soft tissue and therefore cannot rid you of trigger points, the source of so much chronic pain.

Neuromuscular therapy is designed to treat the source of the pain—

the trigger points—in a systematic, drug-free manner. NMT complements and can be used in conjunction with other treatments. It would not be unusual for a neuromuscular massage therapist to consult with a chiropractor, a medical doctor, or an osteopath regarding a client's condition or course of treatment. In some states, chiropractors and medical doctors include neuromuscular therapists on their staff in order to provide an integrated team approach to pain disorders.

Before describing the process of NMT, the next sections of the chapter will provide useful information about trigger points and referred pain. Acquiring this knowledge will help you decide if NMT is a modality you would like to try.

CHARACTERISTICS OF TRIGGER POINTS

Two of the characteristics of trigger points identified and researched by Travell are that they (1) are hyperirritable when compressed, and (2) may refer pain to other areas of the body.

The following example illustrates the hyperirritable nature of trigger points. You are standing in line at the grocery store and a friend comes up behind you and innocently squeezes your shoulder, which happens to contain a trigger point. At the instant of compression, the squeeze, you experience a sudden, sharp pain intense enough to cause you to jump or even cry out.

Trigger points are said to "refer" pain because you may feel the pain not only where your friend inadvertently compressed the trigger point but also at a site distant from the trigger point. In fact, you can experience intense muscle pain at a site that is not the origin of the pain.

In our example, when your friend squeezed your shoulder, the squeeze activated a trigger point in your trapezius muscle, the most common place in the body to have a trigger point. It would not be unusual for the activation of a trigger point in the trapezius muscle to refer or radiate pain up to the back of the ear on the same side, and up to the corner of the eye. Figure 10.1 illustrates the path of the pain from the original site of the trigger point in the trapezius up the head from behind the ear to the corner of the eye.

Each trigger point—and there are many—is associated with a particular repetitive pattern of referred pain.

TYPES OF TRIGGER POINTS

Travell identified several distinct types of trigger points. Knowledge of the way different types of trigger points function can help you understand the nature of your muscle pain. Trigger points may be active or latent, satellite or secondary.

Active Trigger Point

An active trigger point is a focus of hyperirritability in a muscle or its fascia that is painful. It is specific for the muscle. If you have an active trigger point in the muscle or fascia, it will hurt almost all the time, whether you are still or in motion. An active trigger point is like a knot that shortens and weakens the muscle. When an active trigger point is compressed, it will usually refer pain to another site, as exemplified in Figure 10.1. The pain in the referred site is real and can be powerful, even though the pain did not originate there.

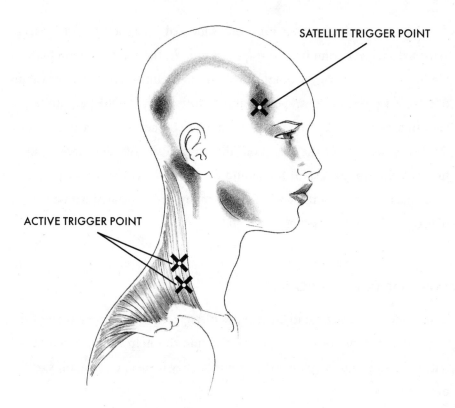

Figure 10.1   A Common Trigger-Point Pattern

Latent Trigger Point

A latent trigger point is a point of hyperirritability in the muscle or the fascia surrounding it that is not always actively painful. It is only painful when palpated or pressed.

Going back to the example of your shoulder being squeezed by your friend at the grocery store, you may not have realized that you had something potentially painful lurking in your shoulder. Another possibility is that you knew from past experience that your shoulder, which does not hurt under ordinary circumstances, would hurt when squeezed, but your friend surprised you, and you did not have the chance to move away. In either case (previous experience with pain to that shoulder or no history of prior pain to that area), it was the squeeze to your shoulder that activated a latent trigger point. With a latent trigger point, your shoulder would not hurt under normal circumstances.

Satellite Trigger Point

A satellite trigger point is a point of hyperirritability in the muscle or its fascia that becomes active because it is in the pain reference zone or path of an active trigger point. The existence and activity of satellite trigger points illustrate how the body acts as a unified system. What happens in one part of the body affects the functioning of other parts of the body.

For example, let's say you have an active trigger point in the trapezius muscle. It will fire a pain pattern that goes up in the back of the neck behind the ear to the corner of the eye—the established pain pattern illustrated in Figure 10.1. Let's say you also happen to have a latent trigger point in the temporalis muscle (in your temple). Because the trigger point in your temple happens to lie in the pain pathway of the trapezius trigger point, it can become active and fire its own pain pattern. In this example, the trigger point in your temple is a satellite trigger point because it happened to be in the pain path of the active trigger point in your trapezius. Now you are suffering from two related pain patterns. It is a case of double trouble.

Secondary Trigger Point

If a trigger point in a particular muscle causes you pain when you exert that muscle, it is natural that you will compensate with other muscles in order to take pressure off the muscle that hurts. As you do this over a prolonged period, latent trigger points in these helper muscles will become active, due to the forced, unnatural movement you impose on them.

For example, if you have an active trigger point in the biceps muscle of your arm, your tendency will be to take pressure off this muscle in order to avoid pain. By doing so, you will force your body into unnatural movements and use neighboring muscles to compensate. Through this process, you may activate a latent trigger point in either of two places: in the brachialis, which lies beneath the biceps, or in the triceps muscle, which lies posterior to the biceps. The trigger points activated in the muscles compensating for your original pain are known as secondary trigger points.

WHY PAIN PATTERNS RECUR

Recurring pain patterns are established through the law of facilitation. According to this law, once a pain pattern is established, it is likely to recur. More specifically, once a pain impulse passes through a certain set of neurons to the exclusion of other neurons, it will tend to take the same course on a future occasion. Every time it takes that path, the resistance will decrease.

Consider this analogy. There is a fresh mound of dirt, and it rains on the mound of dirt. The water runs down the mound, making small crevices for more water to run down. After a few sunny days, the crevices made by the rain are hardly visible. However, the next time it rains, the water will likely take the same path. And every time it rains thereafter, the water will run down the original crevices.

When you have a trigger point that becomes active and painful, that same trigger point will likely make the same pattern of pain every time it is activated. The pattern is predictable for most trigger points.

There are many different reasons for trigger points to become active. Probably the number-one reason is chronic overload of the muscle. If you have a trigger point in your longissimus muscle (one of the main postural muscles that goes all the way down the back from behind the ear), sudden overload of this muscle by lifting without warming up will cause low-back pain. Every time you improperly lift something, you are likely to experience the same pain pattern. This pain pattern will establish itself and recur over time, just like the rainwater in the crevices.

WHAT CAUSES TRIGGER POINTS TO DEVELOP?

Trigger points are caused, in part, by improper circulation. When a muscle or part of a muscle receives an inadequate blood supply, it receives an inadequate supply of oxygen. As a result, the removal of lactic acid and other waste does not occur. As the situation worsens, the tissue becomes ischemic. Ischemia is a lack of blood supply, and the accompanying lack of oxygen, to the muscles and fascia, which causes the affected areas to be oversensitive to touch. An area of soft tissue is considered to be in an ischemic state if less than 5 to 10 pounds of pressure causes a sensation of tenderness.

A number of factors contribute to ischemia in the soft tissue and, in turn, to the development of trigger points. These factors can operate individually or in combination with each other.

Injury

Trigger points can be caused by nerve entrapment or nerve compression resulting from certain types of injuries. Nerve entrapment and compression are conditions in which a bone, cartilage, muscles, or fascia create pressure on a nerve. Treating the soft tissue (muscles and fascia) that causes and maintains the compression can enhance rehabilitation and alleviate pain.

A common injury that causes nerve entrapment by the soft tissues is whiplash, which is the sudden and violent snapping of the neck backward and then forward. This causes your nervous system to react instantly by the tightening of muscles in order to stop the bleeding in the associated tissues. The tightening results in muscular spasms. Well after the bleeding stops, the spasms continue, creating continual or intermittent pressure on nerves—a painful condition. Whiplash is a common problem that will not go away with the mere passage of time. Untreated, it will cause ischemia and trigger points. The trigger points created by whiplash can be treated effectively with neuromuscular therapy.

Mechanical Factors

Mechanical factors perpetuate trigger points in many individuals with chronic pain syndromes. In some cases, the body may be asymmetrical (e.g., one leg shorter than the other), or some parts of the body might stand in disproportion to other parts (e.g., shortened forearms). No one has a perfectly symmetrical or perfectly proportioned body. If the asymmetries and disproportions are relatively small, they are not likely to cause trigger points. However, more significant skeletal asymmetries and greater disproportions of one part to another can be the cause of trigger points.

Other mechanical sources of trigger points include prolonged contraction or prolonged stretching of muscle fibers, for example, due to immobilization in a cast; poor posture; and ergonomic factors, like unsuitable chairs, in the home and workplace. Regarding this last factor, the increasing use of computers at home and at work has caused an enormous increase in trigger points and pain syndromes. This problem can be corrected with the use of proper chairs and chair height.

Internal Factors

Nutritional inadequacies, metabolic and endocrine disorders, chronic infection, and psychological problems are some of the internal factors that can lead to the development of trigger points. Regarding nutritional factors, vitamin C deficiency, for example, can cause postexercise stiffness and a decreased oxygen supply to muscles, resulting in trigger points. Inadequate calcium, potassium, and iron can also lead to dysfunction in the muscle tissue.

In the case of psychological factors, depression and anxiety can contribute to the development of trigger points and chronic physical pain. Individuals who suffer from depression or anxiety disorders tend to hold their bodies in tense positions for prolonged periods. Tension in the face and neck area is common in depressed and anxious individuals. Over time, the tension held in the face and body can cause muscle and fascial tissue to become ischemic and lead to trigger points and pain patterns. Dealing with the physical pain can result in more stress, anxiety, depression, and self-doubt, thus creating a negative mind-body cycle. Travell found that the combination of trigger-point therapy with antidepressant medication has helped many depressed individuals break this negative cycle.

THE PROCESS OF NEUROMUSCULAR THERAPY

The process of neuromuscular therapy can be broken down into two parts: assessment and treatment. Suggestions on how to maintain your gains will also be provided by the practitioner. The client wears a minimal amount of clothing so that the practitioner has maximal access to affected areas. Some of the hands-on work during treatment will require that the skin be dry, whereas other work is more effective with the use of lubrication. As in other massage and bodywork modalities, your comfort and peace of mind are of paramount importance to the practitioner.

Assessment

There are currently no laboratory tests that identify ischemia, trigger points, or the pain patterns caused by them. Only clinical assessment is possible to locate ischemic tissue and trigger points. The clinical assessment performed by the neuromuscular therapist includes taking a detailed history and performing a detailed hands-on examination of the muscles and fascia.

History Taking

When you suffer from chronic pain, several physiological and psychological factors will be explored by the neuromuscular therapist in order to determine and then reduce the causes and intensity of your pain. To promote a full recovery, a variety of factors are addressed during the process of neuromuscular therapy so that all bases are covered. With the goal of comprehensive treatment and full recovery in mind, the practitioner will ask you questions about the history of your pain and factors that may have contributed to it. The topics covered in the history will be those discussed in the previous section of this chapter on the causes of trigger points: injuries, mechanical factors, and internal factors, including nutrition, physical health, psychological functioning, and your use of medication.

In order to obtain a clearer picture of the role of the structure of your body and your posture in the development of trigger points, the practitioner may do a postural analysis. Examining the distortions in your posture can give the practitioner clues as to how you may have created or compensated for your pain. Having this information can help the practitioner show you how to restore proper posture through ergonomics at home and at work and through proper movement. Restoring proper posture helps balance the body and bring it back to homeostasis. Learning how to maintain a state of homeostasis can help you prevent pain patterns from returning.

In addition to answering questions about factors that may have contributed to your chronic pain, you will also be asked in detail about the nature of your pain. For further clarification, you will also be asked to outline, actually draw, the painful areas and pain patterns on a body form chart. By reviewing and refining your actual drawing of the pain pattern, the therapist will be guided as to where to begin treatment.

Manual Examination

Trigger points are located during the assessment through manual palpation and static pressure. The NMT practitioner uses these same hand movements later during the treatment phase, to increase circulation in the trigger-point areas, and to liberate waste products and reduce tension in the affected tissue.

The practitioner may also assess your range of motion in the areas affected by pain. This aspect of the assessment provides information on how the pain has restricted your movement and flexibility, which helps guide the practitioner in establishing treatment.

In some cases, clients begin to experience relief during the assessment phase. It is during the assessment that the practitioner explains to the client the origin of the pain and the course of treatment. This may be the first time a professional has taken your pain seriously and has been able to map out a clear-cut path to the solution. This interaction alone can provide a great deal of mental and emotional relief. Because the mind and the body engage in an ongoing and complex system of communication, physical benefits in the form of release of tension accompany the good news.

Treatment

The progression of treatment in neuromuscular therapy moves from superficial to deeper treatment of the soft tissue. Within the context of neuromuscular work, the techniques of Swedish massage and myofascial release therapy are used for the warming of your muscles to get them ready for deeper treatment.

Communication between the client and practitioner is key in neuromuscular therapy. Because the treatment requires some tolerance for discomfort on the part of the client, the practitioner and client communicate in advance and work within predetermined levels on a discomfort scale. The practitioner may ask you to evaluate your level of discomfort on a scale from 1 to 10 in which 1 indicates no pain at all and 10 is extremely painful. The amount of pressure on a trigger point should be in the 5-to-7 range. If the pressure is too light, the tissue will not respond. If the pressure is too great, the tissue will become even more irritated. Because of the importance of using the correct pressure, communication must be continual throughout each treatment session.

Questions that you might be asked during a session include, Is this area tender? Does the pain refer elsewhere in the body? Where? Is the discomfort lessening in intensity? The practitioner will ask you to express the level of pressure you are experiencing as a number from 1 to 10 so that he or she can adjust the pressure to the 5-to-7 range.

The practitioner will apply pressure to the trigger point or ischemic area for eight to twelve seconds, give the area a brief rest, and then repeat the procedure several times. These compressions push the lactic acid out of the affected areas and, on release, allow blood to enter the areas with fresh nutrients and oxygen. These short, repeated compressions also help break the pain pattern by interrupting the physiopathological reflex circuits. As the work continues, muscle tone becomes normalized, and the nervous system and musculoskeletal system become balanced, restoring homeostasis.

A session of NMT can last anywhere from fifteen minutes to sixty minutes. The number of sessions needed to release the trigger points, break the pain patterns created by them, and ensure that the relief will be long-lasting depends on a number of factors, including the age of the client and the number of trigger points. Another factor is the willingness of the client to make changes that will help maintain gains—for example, using a different height chair for computer work. A rule of thumb is that you should experience at least 50 percent improvement after five sessions. Sometimes, improvement can be achieved sooner.

WHEN NOT TO RECEIVE NMT

All the contraindications for Swedish massage listed in chapter 5 also apply to NMT. Contraindications include (but are not limited to) pregnancy in the first trimester, running a recent fever, active infection, vomiting, nausea, diarrhea, bleeding, and conditions that can lead to blood clotting.

In addition, you should not receive NMT within the first seventy-two hours of an injury or when you are taking pain medication. If you are under medical treatment for a painful condition, consult your medical doctor

Benefits of Neuromuscular Therapy

Relief from chronic pain.

Improved circulation.

Relief from tension and stress.

Better postural patterns.

Greater flexibility and freedom of movement.

Enhanced sense of well-being.

Better understanding of how to prevent relapse.

RELIEF FROM:

* Chronic headaches.

* Low-back pain.

* Eye and ear pain.

* Tinnitus (ringing in the ears).

* Hip and knee pain.

* Elbow/arm/hand pain.

* Sciatica and gluteal pain.

* temporomandibular joint syndrome.

* Carpal tunnel syndrome.

* Cervical whiplash injuries.

* Athletic injuries.

- Rotator cuff injuries.

- Tennis elbow.

- Bulging lumbar and cervical disks.

- Numbness and tingling in the extremities.

- Dizziness, vertigo, and balance problems.

- Swallowing difficulties.

- Body toxicity.

before engaging in neuromuscular therapy, so that your doctor and the NMT practitioner have the opportunity to consult and work as a team in treating your condition.

THE BENEFITS OF NEUROMUSCULAR THERAPY

Neuromuscular therapy relieves chronic pain through locating and eliminating the trigger points that cause the pain. Eliminating the trigger points also eliminates the pain that is referred or radiated to other sites. Most traditional medical doctors do not address trigger points. Many individuals have experienced relief from chronic pain syndromes for the first time when they embarked on a course of NMT.

Some of the pain conditions alleviated by NMT include chronic headaches, low-back pain, eye pain, ear pain and tinnitus (ringing in the ears), hip and knee pain, elbow/arm/hand pain, sciatica and gluteal pain, temporomandibular joint syndrome, and carpal tunnel syndrome. NMT is also effective for the pain associated with cervical whiplash injuries, athletic injuries, rotator cuff injuries, tennis elbow, and bulging lumbar and cervical disks.

NMT also alleviates numbness and tingling in the extremities, dizziness, vertigo, balance problems, and swallowing difficulties. NMT decreases body toxicity, tension, and stress. It improves postural patterns and increases flexibility, freedom of movement, circulation, and your sense of well-being.

EXCELLENT RESULTS IN SIX VISITS

One of our clients came in with hypersensitivity in the lower back, and trigger points and pain-referral patterns in her rotator cuff and erector muscles. After six sessions of NMT, she expressed the following: "I hadn't realized how much pain I was in every day. When I had come to see you, I had learned to live with it. By the second or third session, I was seeing an improvement in how I was feeling every day. I had much more movement in my neck, which would normally stiffen up and stay that way for several days. It was uncomfortable after a day of sitting at a desk to actually get out of my chair and walk home. I was constantly in pain, and I didn't know what to do about it. Now, just coming every couple of weeks has gotten me to the point where I'm not in pain every day. It's just easier to go through everyday tasks and such."

MAXIMIZING AND MAINTAINING THE BENEFITS

Remember that an important aspect of NMT is education regarding the factors that contributed to the development of your trigger points and pain syndrome. It is up to you to maintain the benefits gained through your

NMT experience by correcting the conditions in your internal and external environments that created your chronic pain syndrome.

In order for the receiver to maximize the benefit of NMT, it is important that the giver act as teacher. Understanding the origins of trigger points and learning effective ways of combating and eliminating these painful areas are part of NMT. Homework may be given to the receiver between sessions and, in some cases, as an ongoing maintenance.

The NMT practitioner will explain that trigger points, with their knotlike makeup, actively shorten muscles and their connective tissue. It is not uncommon for the receiver to be given stretching homework between sessions as an adjunct to the therapy for the purpose of expediting the healing process. The giver can show a variety of stretching techniques that are specific to the receiver's affected areas. The purpose of the stretches is to elongate the muscle fibers and connective tissue and eventually reset the proprioceptors (muscle memory) to a more relaxed resting state. These stretching exercises may include passive, active, or active-assisted stretching techniques that are tailored to the receiver's specific needs.

Tennis-ball therapy is another technique that may be recommended between sessions. In this process, the receiver lies on the floor faceup with a tennis ball between his back and the floor and gently rolls around the trigger points in his back. The receiver can modulate the amount of pressure to the trigger points by adjusting his or her weight on the ball. This is a valuable technique for increasing blood flow to the affected areas. The giver may demonstrate the technique so that the receiver has full understanding of the concept and benefit.

Ergonomic changes, such as doing computer work in a chair that is better proportioned to your body, may also be suggested for maximizing and maintaining gains.

Another client reported experiencing chronic pain and poor range of motion in her shoulder. She was unable to lift her arm more than forty-five degrees. After ten sessions of neuromuscular therapy, her condition was significantly improved. She believed that the exercises she was told to do between sessions were an essential part of the treatment and will continue to be essential for maintaining her gains. She considers the treatment plus the exercises "a successful combination."

CHAPTER 11

Shiatsu

The Japanese method of shiatsu is one of the oldest forms of natural healing. The theory underlying this Eastern modality is that by balancing your energy you achieve homeostasis, the steady state that is required to maintain your health and feelings of well-being. Imbalances in energy result in poor health and feeling stressed and fatigued. Although used for treating illness, the focus of shiatsu is more on promoting an internal bodily environment conducive to maintaining good health and preventing disease. Shiatsu is particularly helpful for improving those health states that fall somewhere in between feeling well and feeling ill.

The literal translation of *shiatsu* is "finger pressure." In shiatsu, the practitioner is known as the *giver,* and the client is known as the *receiver*. The type of touch provided by the giver is pressure applied at predetermined, strategic points along the body's surface. The goal of applying pressure at particular points is to unblock and balance the receiver's energy so that the receiver can achieve or maintain homeostasis within the mind-body system. When your mind-body system is in a state of balance, you feel a reduction in stress and an increase in vitality. Beyond the physical, shiatsu is designed to have a positive impact on all levels of functioning, including emotional, mental, and spiritual.

EAST SIDE, WEST SIDE

In the West, shiatsu is the best known form of Eastern bodywork. Although more recently practiced in Japan, shiatsu originated in China. The practice of shiatsu has increased in the West over the past generation more rapidly than any other Eastern bodywork modality. Shiatsu became known in the United States in the 1970s when President Nixon took the first step to bridge the political and cultural gaps between the United States and the Republic of China. Since that time, shiatsu and other Eastern alternative health modalities, including acupuncture and yoga, have become more familiar and widely practiced.

In order to appreciate the science and art of shiatsu, you must first know a little bit about the differences in the Eastern and Western approaches to bodywork and massage. Just as Swedish massage and its derivatives are an outgrowth of Western views of medicine and health, shiatsu is an outgrowth of Eastern views of medicine and health. Swedish massage and shiatsu approach bodywork from different perspectives. The ultimate and shared goal of these representatives of the West and East is to provide a form of therapeutic touch that improves and maintains health and promotes positive feelings and sensations. They differ, however, in both their means of achieving these goals and the theories of health that underlie their divergent techniques.

In the West, being healthy is synonymous with being disease-free. When you are ill, your illness is diagnosed, and medication is prescribed to fight the illness and bring you back into a disease-free state.

In the East, being healthy involves achieving and maintaining homeostasis, a steady, balanced body state. Natural substances and energy-based practices are used to promote and maintain homeostasis.

In Western cultures, being healthy means that all of your individual anatomical parts, including body parts, organs, and internal systems, are functioning well enough that you are symptom-free. Each anatomical part is considered by many professionals separately from the others. In fact, it is not uncommon for one individual to be a patient of a variety of specialists, each with special knowledge about one part of the body (e.g., the foot), one organ (e.g., the heart), and one system (e.g., respiration). No one doctor would necessarily be aware of the patient's condition as a whole.

In Eastern cultures, the person is viewed as a complex mind-body system in which functioning in any one part affects the system as a whole. Being healthy means having sufficient life energy flowing freely through you and all of your internal organs and systems. The life energy, or *ki,* accessed from the universal energy surrounding us, is responsible for our state of health. Maintaining homeostasis and open communication between body and mind are viewed as preventive measures.

The Eastern modalities are based on the premise that a dynamic life force or universal energy animates the mind-body system. This dynamic life force flows throughout the universe and is harnessed by living things—animals, plants, and humans—to maintain life and health. As energy flows through the pathways or meridians in the body, it affects all tissues and organs that control your functioning in daily life.

Energy is invisible. The beliefs that drive Western culture are based more on what can be observed and proven. The concept of energy, something intuitive rather than tangible, is elusive if your mind is trained to view modern science and technology as the bottom line.

The different philosophies of the East and West gave rise to different views on the most effective approaches to preventing and treating illness and injury. In general, prevention is associated more with the East and treatment with the West. In Eastern cultures, the emphasis is on preventing illness and maintaining good health through natural means—for example, by balancing your energy and getting proper nutrition. In Western cultures, the focus is on treatment and cure. These are usually accomplished with medication or surgical procedures that have been tested through the scientific method.

You will see as you read more about the different modalities and their origins that the Eastern and Western approaches are actually compatible and complementary. Together, they present a wider range of paths to your personal goals.

THE ROOTS OF SHIATSU IN
TRADITIONAL CHINESE MEDICINE

Shiatsu is grounded in the theory and practice of traditional Chinese medicine. Although contemporary shiatsu was developed in Japan in the 1800s, its origins date back more than five thousand years to ancient China. It was in these earliest recorded times that health care was preventive in nature.

Acupuncture and Acupressure

One of the earliest forms of Chinese medicine still practiced today is acupuncture. More individuals have used acupuncture than any other medical treatment in history. As in shiatsu, which was developed later, the acupuncturist assesses the energy of the receiver and treats points on the body's surface to release the flow of energy throughout the energy pathways, known as meridians. Unlike the giver of shiatsu, who applies finger pressure to those points, the acupuncturist uses thin needles.

Shiatsu does not use needles or any other kind of instrument (other than the human body). However, because of the commonalities of theory and goals between acupuncture and shiatsu, shiatsu is sometimes referred to as acupressure.

Life Energy

In ancient China, the Taoist priests practiced a form of meditation known as Qi Gong. Qi was considered a vital force that gives life to our bodies and our surroundings. Qi is the energy all around us in the universe. It is available to us and maintains our ability to function. Qi is called *ki* in Japan, *chi* in China, and *prana* in India. It goes by many other names as well, depending on the language of the culture.

The state of your life energy is a direct barometer of the state of your health. If your life energy is plentiful, its elements balanced, and its flow unimpeded, your mind-body system will be homeostatic and humming along. If your life energy is depleted, its elements out of balance, and its flow blocked, you will feel fatigued and be more prone to illness. The purpose of receiving shiatsu is to maintain the balance and flow of your life energy.

Yin and Yang

In traditional Chinese medicine, Qi has two sides—yin and yang. *Yin,* which represents cold and darkness, originally meant "side of the mountain," and *yang,* which represents warmth and light, originally meant "sunside." Thus, on the body, the yang meridians are on the back, because it is the side of the body that normally faces the sun, and the yin meridians are on the front, or shadow side.

The paradox is that even though yin and yang appear to be opposites, they are also complementary. A good analogy is night and day. One is dark and one is light. Both are necessary to complete the day, and you can only appreciate night and day in contrast to each other. You need both yin and yang experiences, and they need to be balanced and in harmony for you to feel complete and function optimally. Thus, in shiatsu, one of the goals of balancing the energy within the mind-body system is to balance yin and yang.

The Five Elements

Built upon the theory of yin and yang is the theory of the five elements of energy—earth, metal, water, wood, and fire. These elements represent the forms that Qi can assume in the physical world. According to traditional Chinese medicine, everything in the physical world is composed of some combination of these elements.

Each element is associated with a season, a color, a sense organ, and internal organs, as depicted in Table 11.1.

In shiatsu, the five elements are used as categories and guidelines for uncovering the nature of each individual's health needs. The tone of the person's skin, how the organs of the body are functioning, physical sensations and symptoms, feelings, dietary habits, the person's stance, presentation,

TABLE 11.1   THE FIVE ELEMENTS OF ENERGY

Element	Season	Color	Sense Organ	Internal Organ
Earth	Late summer	Yellow	Mouth	Spleen and stomach
Metal	Autumn	White	Nose	Lungs and large intestines
Water	Winter	Black	Ears	Bladder and kidneys
Wood	Spring	Blue/ green	Eyes	Liver and gallbladder
Fire	Summer	Red	Tongue	Heart and small intestines

and even the odor of the skin are assessed in the context of yin and yang and the five elements.

The assessment of the receiver's health needs within the context of yin and yang and the five elements guides the giver of shiatsu to the areas along the meridians that require release.

HOW SHIATSU WORKS

Shiatsu prevents disease and maintains health by balancing and unblocking the flow of energy in the meridians. What does that mean?

Meridians are pathways or channels of energy that crisscross the body from one end to the other. They give direction to the flow of energy. Some of the meridians follow the same lines as muscles and blood vessels. There are yin meridians and yang meridians. The system is conceived as having life energy flow through these channels in an organized fashion.

The functions of the meridians include (1) controlling the movement of vital substances (blood, gas, air, and water); (2) connecting the arms, head, and legs with the trunk; (3) controlling the regulation of the organs; and (4) facilitating reciprocal communication inside and outside the body as well as up and down the body.

There are twelve main meridians, each corresponding to an organ for which it is named. Even though the meridians are named for organs, the names of the meridians actually stand for the process of energy flow through that organ rather than for the anatomical part itself. This is an important point, because in Eastern bodywork, the focus is on the flow and balance of energy through the entire person rather than on the functioning of each individual organ.

The free flow of energy through the meridians provides the balance necessary for maintaining good health. Imbalances and blockages may be caused by physical, mental, or even spiritual stressors that create obstructions in the meridians. Stressors are increasingly prevalent and intense in today's society. If the blockages are left untreated, internal systems can eventually break down.

The type of touch used in the shiatsu modality is designed to reduce stress and relieve blockages and imbalances of energy in the meridians. Shiatsu works by maintaining the openness of the meridians mapped out thousands of years ago by releasing constrictions at the pressure points along them.

In addition to applying pressure with the fingers, the giver can choose to touch the receiver's pressure points with his or her palms, thumbs, elbows, or even knees. How and where the pressure is applied depends on the needs of the receiver as assessed by the giver.

As the flow of energy through the meridians becomes unblocked and balanced, all the systems of the body, including the immune system, function more effectively. The support given to your immune system by shiatsu is intended to enhance your own ability to fight disease. According to shiatsu, boosting your immune system and balancing your internal environment are steps that you can take before experiencing the warning signs of impending illness. This concept is at the heart of preventive health care.

EXPERIENCING SHIATSU

A session of shiatsu lasts between sixty and ninety minutes. The experience is different for everyone. Many people experience deep relaxation and renewed vitality. The first shiatsu session begins with an assessment.

Assessment

Through an assessment, the giver determines which pressure points need to be addressed. The giver gathers information and places it within the foundation laid by traditional Chinese medicine, using the concepts of yin and yang and the five elements as a guide.

The assessment is multifaceted. It includes taking a history of your everyday functioning, physical and emotional complaints, current health practices, and nutritional habits and preferences. Another aspect of the assessment is the giver's observation of the receiver. The giver of shiatsu is trained to make special note of the receiver's appearance and movements in order to formulate a treatment plan. For example, someone who appears hunched over, has a yellow skin pallor, and appears tired would have a different profile and might need pressure applied at different points from someone who speaks rapidly and appears sweaty. The assessment indicates to the giver where the energy deficiencies might be located and, therefore, where to apply the pressure, how deeply, and for how long.

Treatment

For the bodywork, the receiver wears loose, comfortable clothing, and no lubrication is applied. It is not needed because there are no gliding strokes and no friction. As the receiver, you place yourself on a futon or comfortable cushion on the floor. Sometimes a massage table is used, but in a lower position than for a traditional massage. For part of the treatment you are asked to lie down, and for other parts you have to sit up (see Figures 11.1 and 11.2).

The only type of touch is one of distinct pressure at varying depths and durations at different points along the surface of the body. These points are located along the meridians. They are standardized and coded so that the giver can apply pressure on those points recorded during the assessment.

Comfortable pressure is applied to the targeted pressure points with the giver's fingers, thumbs, palms, elbows, or knees. All the treatment is manual. No instruments are used.

The touch and process of shiatsu facilitate open communication between giver and receiver. Receptivity to the process can lead to profound effects on the emotional and spiritual levels.

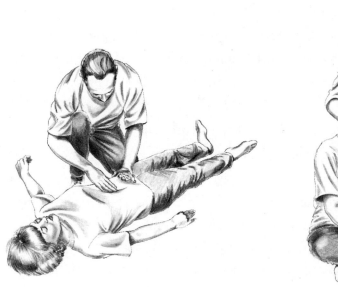

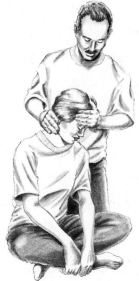

Figure 11.1   Receiving Shiatsu Lying Down   Figure 11.2   Receiving Shiatsu in a
                                                                    Sitting Position

The duration of the session and the frequency of treatment will depend on your needs and preferences. Most individuals feel better immediately after the first session of shiatsu. If you intend to use shiatsu as part of a preventive health plan, you will have to experience it on a regular basis.

THE BENEFITS OF SHIATSU

Shiatsu is a powerful and safe method for accessing the basic sources of life energy available within all of us and promoting the flow of life energy within the body-mind system. The unblocked, natural flow of energy within your system lowers your stress. Many individuals respond to shiatsu with relaxation and renewed vitality.

By unblocking the energy pathways, shiatsu stimulates the activity of the body's vital systems, including the blood and lymph circulatory systems, respiration, the nervous system, and the immune system. By enhancing the functioning of the immune system, shiatsu equips you to prevent and fight disease.

There are many conditions that have been alleviated by shiatsu. These include headaches, migraines, high blood pressure, asthma, bronchitis, sinus conditions, insomnia, fatigue, digestive and elimination disorders, nervous tension, and depression. Shiatsu can alleviate the painful symptoms of arthritis, rheumatism, sore and stiff muscles, sprains, and sports injuries.

Perhaps the biggest benefits of shiatsu are its focus on prevention and the way touch is used to mobilize the body's own healing forces.

Benefits of Shiatsu

Focus on prevention.

Use of touch to mobilize the body's own healing forces.

Enhanced functioning of the immune system.

Promotion of homeostasis within the mind-body system.

Reduced stress.

Feelings of relaxation and renewed vitality.

Increased energy.

STIMULATION OF ACTIVITY IN THE BODY'S VITAL SYSTEMS, INCLUDING:

- Blood and lymph circulatory systems.

- Respiration.

- The nervous system.

- The immune system.

RELIEF FROM:

- High blood pressure.

- Asthma.

- Bronchitis.

- Sinus conditions.

- Fatigue.

- Insomnia.

- Digestive and elimination disorders.

- Nervous tension.

- Headaches.

- Migraines.

- Arthritis.

- Rheumatism.

- Sore and stiff muscles.

- Sprains and sports injuries.

CHAPTER 12

Reflexology

Reflexology is a contemporary form of healing through compression that has been practiced for thousands of years. Although the practice of reflexology is most closely associated with the feet, it is a holistic approach that has benefits for the entire mind-body system. Applying pressure at designated points on the feet, hands, or even ears can create change in all areas of the body.

Like shiatsu, reflexology has its roots in the philosophies and practices of ancient Eastern cultures. Also like shiatsu, a major goal of reflexology is homeostasis, or balance in the mind-body system. Homeostasis promotes harmony and prevents health problems. Whereas in shiatsu the method of balancing the life energy and facilitating homeostasis is by touching strategic points of pressure all over the body, the touch in reflexology is limited primarily to the feet.

Research and case histories have shown that reflexology can provide relief for a wide variety of health problems. This modality was originally developed to balance the internal environment as a means of preventing health problems and enhancing vitality.

THE ORIGINS OF CONTEMPORARY REFLEXOLOGY

Reflexology today is a hybrid of the philosophies and techniques of ancient Oriental medicine and the theories and practices developed in the West. For example, reflexology combines shiatsu's use of pressure points with the Swedish concept that relieving pain by applying direct touch to one area of the body can have a positive impact on other, distant parts of the body.

Ancient illustrations and documents show that the ancient cultures of China, Japan, and Egypt believed that working on the feet was linked to good health. Acupuncture was already commonly practiced, but the application of needles to the feet was considered too painful. Instead of needles, finger pressure was applied to the feet in order to circulate life energy throughout the body. Different areas of the foot were associated with healing different energy centers of the body. Cave drawings in Egypt dating back to 2330 B.C. depict reflexology being given and received.

This modality was introduced to the United States in the early 1900s by Dr. William H. Fitzgerald, a graduate of the University of Vermont. Fitzgerald, calling it *zone therapy,* theorized that there are ten zones located throughout the body, five on the right side and five on the left side. These body zones have corresponding zones in the five toes and five fingers. The zones of the body and the zones of the feet and hands are connected by meridians. These ten meridians are not necessarily the same meridians as those used in shiatsu. Fitzgerald believed and demonstrated that pain relief could be provided by applying the techniques of zone therapy to certain areas of the feet and hands.

In the 1930s, another thread of contemporary reflexology was spun by Eunice Ingham, a physiotherapist who engaged in ten years of intensive research on the specific connections between the feet and the rest of the body. Fitzgerald's zone theory inspired and served as a foundation for her work. Ingham used precise thumb pressure on specific areas of her patients' feet to discover the reaction of each zone of the body to stimulation of different parts of the feet. Based on her recordings of the relationships between tender areas on her patients' feet and the functioning of their organs, glands, and body parts, Ingham mapped out the feet vis-à-vis the body. The method she developed became known as the Original Ingham Method of Reflexology. The term *reflexology* is used because each zone of the body reacts in a reflexive manner to stimulating specific points in the feet.

The descendants of Ingham and students of her method have done further research. Studies of the connections and maps of the feet developed since the pioneering work of Fitzgerald and Ingham show some variations, but the principles remain the same.

THE ZONES OF THE FEET

Reflexologists view the foot as a microcosm of the entire body. Reflex zones in the feet are mapped out into specific areas, each corresponding to a particular body part, organ, or gland. In fact, the map of the foot is a mirror image of the structure of the body. Figures 12.1 and 12.2 illustrate in a general way how the feet have been mapped out. Each area of the foot is labeled according to the body part to which it corresponds.

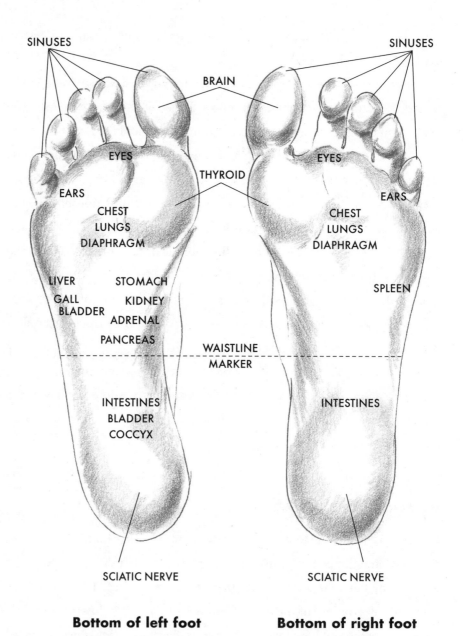

SINUSES

SINUSES

BRAIN

EYES

EYES

THYROID

EARS

EARS

CHEST
LUNGS
DIAPHRAGM

CHEST
LUNGS
DIAPHRAGM

LIVER

STOMACH

SPLEEN

GALL
BLADDER

KIDNEY

ADRENAL

PANCREAS

WAISTLINE
MARKER

INTESTINES
BLADDER
COCCYX

INTESTINES

SCIATIC NERVE

SCIATIC NERVE

Bottom of left foot

Bottom of right foot

Figure 12.1   Zones of the Feet—Bottoms of the Feet

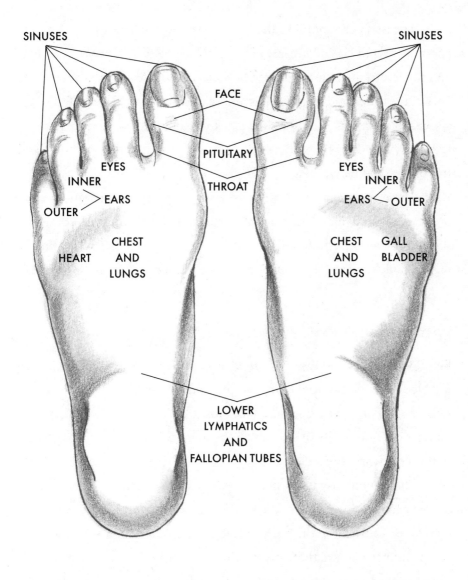

SINUSES

SINUSES

FACE

PITUITARY

THROAT

EYES

INNER

OUTER > EARS

HEART

CHEST
AND
LUNGS

EYES

INNER

EARS > OUTER

CHEST
AND
LUNGS

GALL
BLADDER

LOWER
LYMPHATICS
AND
FALLOPIAN TUBES

Top of left foot

Top of right foot

Figure 12.2   Zones of the Feet—Tops of the Feet

The toes correspond to the head and neck; the balls of the feet to the chest, lung, and shoulder area; the upper arch to the diaphragm, stomach and small intestine; the lower arch to the pelvic and lower intestine; and the heel to the lower body—the pelvis and sciatic nerve. Each outer foot corresponds to each arm, shoulder, hip, leg, knee, and the lower back. The inner foot corresponds to the spine. The ankle area corresponds to the reproductive organs and pelvic area.

These specific areas of the foot are manipulated and compressed in order to promote blood circulation and healing in the corresponding body structure. The compression of the reflex zones is conceptualized as stimulating the body's own healing forces to reduce tension and promote stability.

WHY THE FEET?

Reflexology is a natural way of stimulating the internal organs and increasing blood circulation to all areas of the body through the compression of reflex points on the ears, hands, and, most commonly, the feet. There are a number of reasons why the feet are more often chosen than the hands or ears in this bodywork modality.

The feet are easy to grasp and lend themselves anatomically to receiving reflexology. Having the feet worked on allows the receiver to sit in a relaxed, comfortable position. The feet contain more than seven thousand nerve endings and are therefore sensitive to touch and have many connections throughout the nervous system. These features enhance the connection to the zones and systems of the body.

The feet are also the best choice for reflexology because the feet themselves are more prone to strain than the hands and ears because of the support they provide to the entire body. In addition, because of the location of the feet and the impact of gravity, your feet and ankles are more likely to accumulate toxins than are your hands or ears. A related issue for the feet is their distance from the heart, making them a target for less optimal circulation of blood and lymph. The accumulation of waste and toxins in the lower extremities and feet can cause edema, or swelling. Compression applied directly to the feet can relieve the impact of strain, improve circulation, and promote the elimination of waste products that have settled there.

Even though the feet are the most common target area in this treatment modality, reflexology is not simply a foot massage. Rather, it is a method for healing dysfunction and pain in the whole body through the compression of the different areas of each foot.

EXPERIENCING REFLEXOLOGY

As the receiver, you are asked to remove your socks and shoes. No other clothing is removed. As a courtesy to the giver, the receiver's feet should be clean for the session. The giver might apply light oil or olive oil, light powder or cornstarch, or nothing at all to the feet during the reflexology session. The session can last anywhere from twenty to sixty minutes. For the duration of the session, the receiver sits in a reclined position in a comfortable, padded chair.

The giver of reflexology will work systematically by applying finger and thumb pressure at varying depths and durations to the zones of your feet. By compressing areas over the entire foot—bottom, side, top, and ankles—the giver can determine the tender areas that need to be the focus of treatment. The giver will apply firm pressure in order to relieve the tension in these tender areas. While performing reflexology, the giver's compression of your feet will stay within the parameters of your comfort and resistance.

When the session is over, you will most likely feel relaxed and energized. If you have a specific health complaint that was alleviated in the reflexology session, you can discuss with the giver a schedule for further remediation of the problem and prevention of recurrence.

IS REFLEXOLOGY EFFECTIVE?

The value of reflexology for preventing, fighting, and healing illness has been studied extensively all over the world. Because of its roots in traditional Chinese medicine, the majority of the research on the effectiveness of reflexology has been performed in China. The intent of research on reflexology is not to claim this modality as a substitute for medical treatment. Rather, it is being explored as an adjunct to treatment and as an option to consider under the appropriate circumstances.

Research on reflexology has addressed its health benefits for the general population as well as its application in the workplace for reducing stress, illness, and absenteeism. Researchers have examined the impact of reflexology on many health problems (see "Benefits of Reflexology" at the end of this chapter).

In 1996, the *China Reflexology Symposium Report* of the China Reflexology Association reviewed and analyzed 8,096 clinical cases involving foot reflexology. This massage project was headed by Dr. Wang Liang who reported that foot reflexology was effective in treating more than 93 percent of the disorders reviewed.

Research Areas in Reflexology

Anemia	Cerebral palsy	Hiccough
Angina	Cholesterol	Hypertension
Ankle sprain	Constipation	Insomnia
Anxiety	Diabetes	Muscle pain
Arthritis	Diarrhea	Pneumonia
Asthma	Enuresis	Rheumatoid arthritis
Bell's Palsy	Gout	
Blood circulation	Gynecological disorder	Stiff neck
Bronchitis		Toothache
Cataracts	Headaches	Urinary disorders

Liang divided the results of the review into three categories:

1. Cure or significant and lasting effect.
2. Some improvement or effect that includes partial disappearance of symptoms, but recurrence without treatment.
3. Insignificant or no effect.

Of the 8,096 cases studied, 45 percent showed some improvement. More than 48 percent showed foot reflexology to be either a cure or significantly effective. In about 6 percent of the cases, reflexology had no effect.

The health problems for which foot reflexology was found to be effective include vertigo, upper respiratory tract infection, flu, chronic constipation, gastroenteritis, and type 2 diabetes. Research findings suggest that reflexology could play a role in lowering cholesterol. It also looks like foot reflexology can decrease free radicals in the blood. The efficient elimination of free radicals will help restore balance, eliminate toxins, and fortify the immune system, thereby equipping you to prevent and fight disease more effectively.

OTHER BENEFITS OF REFLEXOLOGY

The main benefits of reflexology are the relief of nervous tension, improved circulation, and the restoration of homeostasis and balance in the body. Reflexology benefits the mind-body system by preparing it to prevent and fight illness. It does this by balancing the energy and stimulating the immune system.

Reflexology reduces both the physical and mental components of stress. After a session of reflexology, many individuals concentrate better and work more efficiently. They feel renewed. The effectiveness of reflexology for reducing stress, improving attitudes, and increasing productivity has led some companies to provide regular reflexology treatments during the day in the workplace. Reflexology is a benefit not only to the employees but also to the employers who want to use it to promote morale and as a preventive health measure for reducing illness and absenteeism. Because reflexology is applied to the feet, it is easy to implement in the workplace.

Another advantage of the application of bodywork only to the feet or hands is that no touching or pressure is applied directly to tender or injured body parts. In addition, there are some cases in which the direct stimulation of the lymph or other bodily fluids can spread a systemic problem, which makes some forms of bodywork contraindicated. Reflexology is a safe modality because the stimulation of internal fluids and systems is indirect, emanating from the nerve endings and muscles in the feet.

In addition, if you feel uncomfortable with full-body massage or bodywork, you can still derive many of the benefits with only your feet being exposed or touched.

There has been extensive research on reflexology and its application to a wide variety of health problems. For individuals with no particular health problem, who do not feel particularly stressed, and who are able to maintain balance and homeostasis through other means, reflexology can still provide benefits. Many individuals who receive this modality experience a satisfying sense of relaxation coupled with increased vitality and alertness. These are the ingredients for creative thinking and productivity in anything you decide to pursue.

Benefits of Reflexology

Relief of stress and nervous tension.

Enhanced relaxation.

Increased vitality and alertness.

Enhanced creativity and productivity.

Improved circulation.

(continued on next page)

Restoration of homeostasis and the balance of energy in the mind-body system.

Stimulation of the immune system.

Prevention of illness.

Absence of direct pressure to injured body parts.

No danger of spreading systemic illnesses.

RELIEF FROM:

* Vertigo.

* Asthma.

* Upper respiratory tract infection.

* Flu.

* Chronic constipation.

* Gastroenteritis.

* Type 2 diabetes.

* Kidney stones.

* Muscular pain.

* Sciatica.

* Pain due to injury.

* Headaches.

Gentle Touching with Profound Results

The Trager Approach

Manual Lymph Drainage

Craniosacral Therapy

The Rosen Method

I t would be a mistake to equate gentle touch with mild results. The modalities included in this section represent diverse approaches that have in common subtle, gentle touch with pervasive, significant positive changes in physical health and feelings of well-being.

CHAPTER 13

The Trager Approach

The Trager Approach is a unique form of mind-body education that teaches your mind to trigger a relaxation response in your muscles and fascia through the application of light, gentle strokes. This approach is designed to help you move your body more freely and with less effort.

HOW TRAGER DIFFERS FROM OTHER APPROACHES

The Trager Approach is not massage. In fact, this bodywork approach is very different in intent and style from any bodywork approach that uses direct manual pressure to release muscle tension and tight fascia. Trager is light and seems effortless. The lightness and subtlety of the Trager Approach in no way detract from its effectiveness in alleviating muscle tension. In fact, it is a very powerful modality.

The manner in which the body is manipulated in the Trager Approach is not considered a technique or a method. Although there are guiding principles, there is no standard set of procedures in the Trager Approach, as there are in most massage and bodywork modalities.

In other modalities, the positive impact of touch on mental functioning is a side benefit. In the Trager Approach, improved mental functioning through touch is central to the process. Gentle strokes and rocking motions are applied to your body in order to communicate tactile messages to your mind, specifically your brain and nervous system. The result is that your mind does the releasing of bodily tension for you.

THE BODY AS A CONDUIT TO THE UNCONSCIOUS

The theory underlying the Trager Approach is that pain, muscle spasms, tightness, and blocked movement originate in and are maintained by the chemistry and neurological circuits of the mind. Through life experience, the mind receives negative messages that train it to hold on tightly to the muscles, creating tension, rigidity, restricted movement, and pain. Over time, unconscious blockages develop and become habitual, preventing the mind from signaling the body to let go of the muscle tension. As the blockages in the mind-body feedback loop become more deeply entrenched, dysfunctional movement patterns are created. We get so used to these patterns that they seem normal to us. When this happens, chronic pain can become a way of life.

Because these holding patterns are at an unconscious level and because there is an increasing failure of the body and mind to communicate in a healthy way, the roots of the dysfunctional patterns become difficult to access and change on our own. We cannot simply will ourselves to relax.

The Trager Approach is designed to help you release your mental hold on your muscles so that you can free them of spasm and pain. The Trager practitioner uses strokes intended to signal the part of your mind that controls your body to let go of the tension held in your soft tissue. The touch communication creates a feedback loop from body to mind and back to the body again. Through touch, psychophysiological blockages in the mind and the body are released, promoting an increase in energy, deep relaxation, release of muscular tension, relief from chronic pain, and the integration of body and mind.

According to Betty Post, a certified Trager practitioner, the amount of pressure applied during a Trager session depends on the boundaries of the person being treated. The practitioner is trained not to push past the client's point of resistance. Post and other Trager practitioners perceive little value in using techniques that involve applying strong pressure to the tense soft tissue, because only temporary relief can be gained in this way. Post believes that, although other modalities can provide temporary relief from muscle tension, the holding patterns in the mind will remain. In fact, applying strong pressure against the resistance of the muscle tissue will prevent the releasing tactile messages from being received, and the mind will hold on with equal resistance, creating the opposite of the desired effect.

As the mind receives the input through the practitioner's touch, endorphins are released from the brain, and long-standing holding patterns are broken. The result is decreased muscle tension, greater ease of movement, a pleasurable body state, and an increased capacity for communication between body and mind.

Thus, the goal of the Trager Approach is to communicate with your mind through touching your body and to unblock the pathways between mind and body. Cumulative and long-lasting results can be achieved through the focus on conveying new messages to that part of the unconscious mind that signals the muscles throughout the body to tense up or relax. Through revising unconscious painful mind-body patterns, the Trager Approach clears the way for greater mental clarity, long-lasting pain relief, increased flexibility and freedom of movement, and the reduction of aches, muscle spasms, and stress.

THE LIFE AND WORK OF MILTON TRAGER

The development of the Trager Approach was not planned. Rather, it evolved naturally because of the special talents of one man—Milton Trager, M.D. A full appreciation of the Trager Approach can be achieved only by taking a look at the history of Milton Trager's life and career.

Trager was born in Chicago in 1908. As a teenager, he was in training as a boxer when he realized that the real gift in his hands was their power to heal rather than to fight. He gave his trainer a massage based purely on intuition as to what to do, and his trainer was amazed at the effectiveness of Trager's touch. When Trager went home, he offered to work manually on his father's unrelenting sciatica, eased his pain substantially after just one session, and then completely freed his father from symptoms after two more sessions.

At this point, Trager decided to protect his hands. He quit boxing and worked as an acrobat and a dancer. When he was only age nineteen, he used his hands to help a sixteen-year-old polio victim walk again. After that experience, he sought out people who found no relief for their problems through conventional approaches.

After receiving formal training, he worked as a physical therapist during World War II in the navy, and then on individuals with postwar neuromuscular disorders. At age forty-one, he wanted to become a medical doctor in order to legitimatize his hands-on work. His determination to find a school to accept him as a medical student at his age led him to the University Autonoma de Guadalajara in Mexico.

While attending medical school as a specialist in polio, Trager applied his hands-on approach to the body of a four-year-old victim of polio who had been paralyzed from the waist down since she was age two. After one forty-minute session, the girl could move her foot and twitch her leg in four directions. His special talents stunned both the medical and religious communities. Over the years he discovered that individuals with less serious physical disorders also benefited from his approach to bodywork.

After receiving a medical degree in 1955, Trager did his internship in Hawaii, where he and his wife settled for the next eighteen years. He developed a private practice in general medicine and physical rehabilitation. It was also in the 1950s that he was among the few Americans initiated in Transcendental Meditation by the Maharishi Mahesh Yogi. Trager applied what he learned about meditation to his approach in bodywork.

It was not until the 1970s that Trager began to realize his methods could be taught to others. His teaching began tentatively with one therapist to help one particular patient. In 1975, he did his first public demonstration at Esalen Institute, where he met Betty Fuller, a group leader. She was so impressed with the relief she obtained through his gentle approach that she persuaded him to create a training program. Trager and Fuller founded the Trager Institute in Mill Valley, California. Trager eventually closed his private practice in order to devote his full energies to training students.

Currently, there are more than one thousand certified practitioners throughout the world. There are thirteen qualified instructors who travel throughout the world to provide training programs in the Trager Approach. Trager worked actively as a teacher and practitioner until his death in 1997.

EXPERIENCING THE TRAGER APPROACH

There are two distinct but related processes involved in the Trager Approach. The first process is the phase in which the practitioner performs the gentle hands-on table work known as Psychophysical Integration. The second process, Mentastics, involves learning movements that allow you to explore self-healing. Using the Mentastics on your own will help you maintain and expand on the gains made during table work.

Psychophysical Integration

Psychophysical Integration is received while the client lies under a sheet or light blanket on a padded bodywork table. During these sessions, the client wears anything ranging from comfortable clothing to just underwear, depending on his comfort level. No oil is used because there are no strokes in which friction is a major factor. A session lasts between sixty and ninety minutes. There is no set series of sessions. Because it takes time to undo old patterns and reestablish healthy communication between body and mind, it makes sense that more than one session would be helpful in achieving the desired results.

As the client, you lie comfortably supported on the cushioned table. The Trager practitioner moves each part of your body gently through motions, including rocking, rolling, stretching, light compression, and vibration. The practitioner takes your joints through their range of motion at a level that goes no further than your natural resistance, allowing you to experience moving freely and comfortably within your pain-free range. The back is an important area of focus. Rather than using a massage motion, the practitioner lets the client appreciate the length of the back and its relationship to the rest of the body.

While applying the strokes, the practitioner will be listening for and sensing feedback to find your boundaries of resistance, flexibility, and range of motion. The practitioner will use this feedback to select the movements and pressure best tailored to your needs. No two Trager sessions are alike, because no two people are alike, and each person's needs differ from session to session.

Effective listening for and sensing of your needs is achieved by the Trager practitioner, who is trained to enter into a mental state known as hook-up, which is an active form of meditation. Achieving this state is considered essential to the process, because doing so enables the practitioner to relax fully, become more intuitively attuned to your body's responses, and select the strokes that will work best for you. According to the Trager Approach, the practitioner's mental state and pleasant feelings will be communicated and transmitted to the client.

All the touching will be gentle and nonintrusive. The strokes used in the Trager Approach do not put pressure on muscle tissue or fascia. Tight areas will be approached with light touch, and nothing will be forced. In fact, when resistance is encountered, the practitioner's strokes will become lighter, not deeper. The hands of the practitioner will communicate the lightness and freedom that your body wants to feel. Even though the strokes are light, the effect can be profound.

These light, soft touches and gentle rocking movements are used by the practitioner to lull the client's mind and body into releasing muscle tension. Your mind will begin to send messages of release to your muscles, allowing them to relax. As you willingly give up muscular and mental control, you will sink slowly and pleasurably into a deep state of relaxation. As you continue to move more deeply into mental and physical relaxation, blockages will be opened, and your mind and body will become better connected. Your mind will learn how to signal your muscles to relax with less help from the practitioner.

Mentastics

After the hands-on portion of the session, the client is given instruction in the use of Mentastics, or mental gymnastics. *Mentastics,* which is a term coined by Trager, are mind-body exercises and a system of movement sequences taught to the client by the Trager practitioner.

Different from stretching or routine exercise, Mentastics are playful, creative movements that use gravity as your friend. You release tension by surrendering your weight to the force of gravity—for example, by letting your arms hang down and swing gently. Some individuals who experience the table work invent their own Mentastics routine.

The purpose of doing Mentastics is to maintain and add to the gains achieved through the Psychophysical Integration session. Mentastics help re-create and enhance the ease of movement and sense of lightness enjoyed during the session. Engaging in these exercises is at least as important as the table work in keeping communication open between mind and body.

CONDITIONS TREATED SUCCESSFULLY
WITH THE TRAGER APPROACH

Although Milton Trager was a medical doctor and the Trager Approach can be used to alleviate the pain and restricted-movement symptoms of a variety of illnesses, the Trager Approach is not a form of medical treatment. It is an alternative approach.

Trager's focus during his long career was on applying his approach to severe neuromuscular disturbances that did not respond adequately to conventional medical approaches. The Trager Approach has been used with amazing success for the alleviation of the symptoms of seriously debilitating medical conditions, like polio, paralysis, muscular dystrophy, multiple sclerosis, and Parkinson's disease.

Trager realized, however, through experience with a wide variety of clients, that his approach could be applied with success to less severe, more common problems that many individuals experience in daily life. These include asthma, carpal tunnel syndrome, migraine headaches, chronic pain syndromes, restricted and painful movement, muscle tension, muscle spasms, poor posture, depression, and chronic stress. Back pain is considered a specialty of this bodywork modality.

OTHER BENEFITS

In addition to treating the symptoms of specific, diagnosable conditions, the Trager Approach has other benefits. Individuals experiencing the Trager Approach have reported a wide range of mind-body benefits, including a feeling of calmness, a greater connection with the self, an enjoyment of the body, renewed vitality, ease of movement, increased mental clarity, and greater emotional freedom. Some clients experience the renewed integration of body and mind as a sense of balance and inner peace.

Benefits of the Trager Approach

Calmness of the mind.

Greater connection with the self.

Enjoyment of the body.

Renewed vitality.

Ease and flexibility of movement.

Increased mental clarity.

Greater emotional freedom.

A sense of balance and inner peace.

Improved athletic performance.

RELIEF FROM PAIN AND MOVEMENT PROBLEMS ASSOCIATED WITH SEVERE NEUROMUSCULAR CONDITIONS, INCLUDING:

* Polio.

* Paralysis.

* Muscular dystrophy.

* Multiple sclerosis.

* Parkinson's disease.

RELIEF FROM THE SYMPTOMS OF MORE COMMON PROBLEMS, INCLUDING:

* Asthma.

* Carpal tunnel syndrome.

* Migraine headaches.

* Chronic pain syndromes.

* Restricted and painful movement.

* Muscle tension.

* Muscle spasms.

* Poor posture.

* Depression.

* Chronic stress.

* Back pain (considered a specialty).

TRAGER FOR ATHLETES

As discussed earlier in this chapter, Milton Trager was an athlete and a dancer. It was natural that he incorporate his grace and athleticism into his approach. Many professional athletes, as well as average individuals who enjoy sports or bodybuilding, have benefited from the Trager Approach.

What the Trager Approach does for athletes is multifaceted. Undergoing the Trager Approach (both table work and Mentastics) has helped athletes improve their mental focus, remain centered when tired or falling short of a goal, connect bodily movement to what the mind wants the body to do, relax tense muscles, increase the flexibility of both body and mind, and gain better emotional control. A growing number of trainers are encouraging their clients to participate in the Trager Approach in order to help them avoid burnout, to develop better endurance, and to get the edge.

The sports to which the Trager Approach has been applied successfully include running, bicycling, swimming, tennis, and golf. Golfers report that the softening of muscles in the shoulder area results in improved putting.

Benefits of the Trager Approach for Athletes

Improved mental focus.

Maintenance of centeredness when tired or falling short of a goal.

Connection of bodily movement to what the mind wants the body to do.

Relaxation of tense muscles.

Increased flexibility of both body and mind.

Better emotional control.

Better physical and mental endurance.

Prevention of burnout.

BE OPEN ABOUT MEDICAL CONDITIONS
AND MEDICATIONS

Although the Trager Approach is safe for most individuals because of the gentle nature of the strokes, there are a few contraindications. If you have a medical condition, disclose the details to the Trager practitioner in case the approach needs to be more carefully tailored. The practitioner may advise you to consult your physician first.

CHAPTER 14

Manual Lymph Drainage

Manual lymph drainage, or MLD, is a therapeutic massage modality with a specialized goal: improving the functioning of the lymphatic system by stimulating the flow of lymph. Although improving the functioning of any system of the body could benefit most of us, MLD is particularly designed to help individuals with dysfunction in the efficiency of their lymphatic system.

MASSAGE AND THE CIRCULATION OF BODILY FLUIDS

In order to appreciate the mechanisms and benefits of manual lymph drainage, you must first understand that a feature most massage modalities have in common is their positive impact on the circulation of fluids throughout the body. Improved circulation of the fluids in the various systems of the body promotes both physical and mental health.

As discussed in chapter 5, Swedish massage is known for improving blood circulation, which helps warm the extremities and promotes feelings of vitality and well-being. MLD is a special modality derived from Swedish massage. Rather than focusing on the circulation of blood, MLD consists of a set of guiding principles and strokes targeted at improving the circulation of a different bodily fluid—namely, lymph.

The proper flow of lymph is important in maintaining your health for several reasons: (1) It helps the body eliminate toxins and swelling; (2) it facilitates the purification and regeneration of body tissue; (3) it helps maintain the healthy functioning of your internal organs; and (4) it promotes the functioning of the immune system. An unobstructed, efficient lymphatic system also allows for homeostasis, a steady, balanced state of the body's complex chemistry. When your body is out of homeostasis, you feel the sense of imbalance in many subtle and not-so-subtle ways.

For some individuals, inefficiency of the lymphatic system can lead to lymphedema, the overaccumulation of lymph in parts of the body, often in the extremities, creating swelling. MLD can alleviate the swelling caused by lymphedema.

The specialized massage strokes of MLD were designed to address the needs of individuals who suffer from lymphedema. These strokes were developed for the express purpose of stimulating the flow of lymph so that waste products and toxins can be more effectively and efficiently eliminated from the internal environment of the body.

THE IMPORTANCE OF THE LYMPHATIC SYSTEM
AND THE FLOW OF LYMPH

Manual lymph drainage, also called Vodder lymph drainage (discussed later in this chapter), assists in the functioning of the lymphatic system by improving the circulation of lymph as it flows throughout this system's network of ducts, vessels, and capillaries. The lymphatic system, which is almost as extensive as the blood circulatory system, identifies and rids the body of disease-producing microorganisms, which are absorbed and destroyed by the lymph.

Lymph is a clear, colorless fluid that flows throughout these vessels at a rate slower than blood. It carries with it excess water, various waste products, and foreign substances that should be eliminated from the body for optimal functioning. The unobstructed flow of lymph allows for greater effectiveness and efficiency in the removal of excess fluid, protein, wastes, and toxins.

The body functions better and people feel better when not carrying around excess waste products. Individuals with healthy lymphatic systems report more physical and mental energy and an increase in feelings of well-being.

Proper functioning of the immune system is dependent on the functioning of the lymphatic system. The immune system produces lymphocytes, white blood corpuscles, which play a critical role in healing wounds and fighting disease. These strong, healing blood cells are transported by the lymph. The ability of these cells to reach their destination is impeded by the inefficient flow of lymph.

Poor lymph circulation can result in the increased retention of waste products in the tissues of the body. This can make you feel tired, even exhausted. It adversely affects your metabolism and creates an internal environment more prone to disease.

LYMPHEDEMA

When the molecules of waste products become too large to be absorbed by the lymphatic system, they cannot be destroyed. When this problem gets out of control, the individual can develop lymphedema, a special form of edema.

Edema is swelling caused by the abnormal accumulation of fluid in the cells, tissues, and cavities of the body. In the case of lymphedema, the excess fluid contains dead protein, which, if allowed to accumulate indefinitely without treatment, could lead to chronic swelling, pain, and disfigurement of those areas affected. Lymphedema can also result in unhealthy changes in the tissues and cells of the body, which can lead to disease. If the legs or feet are affected by lymphedema, mobility can become impaired.

More than 3 million Americans suffer from lymphedema. Some individuals develop this condition after certain physically traumatic events, such as surgery and radiation for various types of cancer, including breast and prostate. In such instances, the lymphedema would be called secondary, because it would be a result of, or secondary to, something else—for example, the physical assault to the system caused by mastectomy. Others are diagnosed with primary edema, in which case the cause is congenital or unknown and the symptoms can emerge at any point.

If the lymphedema (whether primary or secondary) is chronic, treatment should be received on an ongoing basis. Without treatment, lymphedema worsens. The swelling increases in affected areas. The movement in the joints can become increasingly restricted and painful. In addition to the discomfort factor, lymphedema can also be a serious health concern. Because the stagnant protein lymph fluid provides a friendly environment for the growth of bacteria and fungi, infections can develop. Some of these infections can be severe.

Although lymphedema cannot be cured, the symptoms and discomfort can be alleviated. The affected part of the body can be restored to closer to normal size and shape, and the condition can be kept from worsening.

Manual lymph drainage massage has been shown to be effective in alleviating the symptoms of lymphedema. The practice of MLD includes movements specifically designed to stimulate vessels that reside near the lymph vessels, to carry the overloaded lymph away from the edema site. Please keep in mind that MLD is not intended as a substitute for other treatments that your doctor might recommend. Individuals who suffer from lymphedema or other medical conditions should consult their physician before undergoing MLD.

MLD VERSUS SWEDISH MASSAGE

To the untrained eye, MLD massage could easily be mistaken for Swedish massage, on which it is founded. But, while both of these modalities share the goal of improving the flow of lymph, Swedish massage has other goals as well, including improving blood circulation and promoting relaxation. Manual lymph drainage, on the other hand, is *specifically* designed to improve the flow of lymph. It is an area of specialization that requires training beyond Swedish massage.

Because a major focus of Swedish massage is to improve blood circulation, the therapists' strokes are long and flowing. Not much pumping is necessary in Swedish massage because the circulation of blood is already stimulated and maintained by the body's internal pump—the heart. However, there is no internal pump for lymph. The specialized strokes of the trained MLD massage therapist compensate, in a sense, for the lack of an internal lymph pump by working like an external pump for the regulation of the flow of lymph.

THE PROCESS AND EXPERIENCE OF MLD

MLD is experienced as a gentle massage modality. As the client, you lie down on a padded massage table under a sheet with your clothing removed, just as you would in Swedish massage. The massage begins at the base of the neck. The neck treatment is performed first to clear out the main pathways. Then the arms, legs, trunk, and finally the back are massaged.

During the MLD process, only the skin is moved by the practitioner's touch, because 40 percent of the body's lymph resides in these superficial layers. Systematic rhythmic and pumping strokes unblock lymphatic flow and increase the elimination of bodily wastes, toxins, and pathogens. Activated by massage, lymph vessels may carry up to ten times more waste than they normally do.

The practitioner of this modality uses light, slow, repetitive strokes specifically designed to boost the circulation of lymph. The touches are gentle, rhythmic, and pumping, all following the direction of the flow of lymph. The MLD practitioner generally starts at the base of the client's neck before moving to the extremities.

The practitioner alternates gentle pressure and release as a means of opening and closing the lymph valves. Pumping motions, with the practitioner's palms pressing toward the center of the body, are also applied to move the lymph along. Circular movements are used as well. Some of the circular strokes are made by the practitioner's fingers repetitively working in the same area; other circular strokes are more like spiraling motions, moving outward. Circular strokes are typically applied to the neck, face, and lymph nodes. These types of motions are intended to gently encourage the flow of lymph, rather than to force it. You, as the client, should not experience any pain as part of this process.

The precise amount of pressure, the speed of the movements, and the length of time used to massage a particular part of the body depend on the needs of each client. The skilled MLD practitioner uses feedback from the feeling and responsiveness of the skin and soft tissue to determine which movements are best applied to a particular person at different points in treatment. Clients are advised to lie quietly after the massage until they feel comfortable getting up and moving around.

Many individuals who have experienced this massage modality report that it makes them feel stimulated and energized. The positive effects are maintained for varying lengths of time after one session. The more precisely the techniques of MLD are applied, the better the results. However, even the most skilled practitioner cannot prevent lymphedema from recurring. If you suffer from chronic lymphedema, more than one lymph drainage massage will be necessary to maintain gains. Otherwise, the lymphatic system will become increasingly inefficient, and problems will recur without treatment.

BENEFITS OF MLD

Manual lymph drainage is used primarily to alleviate conditions characterized by poor lymph flow, such as edema and lymphedema, conditions which can result from cancer, treatments for cancer, and radical mastectomy. This modality has been found to be more effective for alleviating the symptoms and discomfort of these conditions than mechanized methods or diuretic drugs.

MLD massage has also been shown to be effective in improving the functioning of the immune system. It does this by producing lymph cells that help heal wounds and fight infections and by stimulating the vessels that carry these cells to the relevant body tissue and organs.

Specific benefits include the relief of pain, swelling, and fibrosis in postmastectomy and postamputation patients, the alleviation of both primary and secondary lymphedema, stronger immunity against infection and systemic disease, and the reestablishment of balance within the body's complex chemistry.

The benefits of MLD are not limited to individuals with health problems. MLD can also benefit healthy individuals as a cleansing process that helps eliminate accumulated toxins from the body. MLD also increases energy and vitality as it calms and relaxes.

THE VODDERS

The massage practice of manual lymph drainage was developed in the 1930s by Dr. Emil Vodder and Estrid Vodder, husband and wife. The Vodders were from Denmark and worked as physical therapists in France. They studied the

Benefits of MLD

Relief from the symptoms and discomfort of primary
lymphedema, which is congenital and whose causes
may be unknown.

Relief from the symptoms and discomfort of lymphedema,
pain, swelling, and fibrosis that are secondary to
cancer, postcancer treatments, or radical mastectomy.

Improved flow of lymph throughout the lymphatic system,
thereby facilitating the elimination of toxins and wastes
from body tissues.

Improved functioning of the immune system in fighting
infection and disease.

Restoration of the complex chemistry of the body to
homeostasis.

Increased energy and vitality.

Enhanced relaxation.

lymphatic system and discovered that the movement and flow of lymph could be stimulated and enhanced through specialized touch consisting of a series of light, rhythmic manipulations. Through the application of these strokes to the needs of their physical therapy patients, the Vodders developed and coined *manual lymph drainage,* a systematic approach to treating the lymphatic system through specialized touch techniques.

After World War II, the Vodders returned to their native Denmark.

They established the Dr. Vodder Center in Copenhagen, taught MLD to European therapists, and trained others to teach this massage modality. The Vodders designated Hildegard and Gunther Wittlinger as their successors and authorized them to teach the original Dr. Vodder MLD method. In 1971, the Wittlingers established the Dr. Vodder School and Clinic in Walchsee, Austria. The facility has become an internationally recognized center for the study of MLD. Other centers were established in Europe in the 1970s. In 1976, MLD was recognized officially by the German Society of Lymphology. The Wittlingers have taught extensively in the United States and Canada, clearly establishing the Dr. Vodder method as the best and most well-known lymphatic drainage technique.

Although widely practiced in Europe, MLD massage has not been as popular in North America. However, its popularity and availability in the United States and Canada are increasing rapidly. To meet the growing need for trained MLD practitioners in the United States and Canada, the Dr. Vodder School–North America was established in 1994 according to the stringent standards of its European counterparts.

THE TRAINED MLD PRACTITIONER

To perform manual lymph drainage, the practitioner must have special training in this modality, including a thorough knowledge of anatomy and of the lymphatic system. The massage movements in MLD are precise and should be applied in the way originally taught by the Vodders.

The Dr. Vodder School–North America in Victoria, British Columbia, is the only school in North America authorized to teach the original Vodder method of manual lymph drainage. There are approximately 340 certified Dr. Vodder manual lymph drainage therapists in North America today. The demand is growing because of the effectiveness of MLD in treating lymphedema. The types of professionals trained at this prestigious school include nurses, occupational therapists, and medical doctors.

According to the school's course catalog, many Vodder-trained MLD therapists and students are members of the North American Vodder Association of Lymphatic Therapy (NAVALT). This professional, nonprofit association was founded in 1992 and is dedicated to the advancement of the Dr. Vodder method of manual lymph drainage through high standards, education, and research.

A REWARDING PROFESSION

Kim Buckalew, a massage therapist, became interested in specializing in manual lymph drainage massage after a job interview in which she was shown before and after pictures of lymphedema. She said at the time, "Wow, how rewarding." After five years of doing more conventional massage, she received training in manual lymph drainage at the Academy of Lymphatic Studies in Princeton, New Jersey. Most of her clients have had cancer. Kim evaluates each person as an individual and plans a schedule of treatment that ends with a maintenance schedule.

Kim emphasizes the importance of self-care for improvement and maintenance: "I teach them to take care of themselves. There are things they can do at home—bandaging at night, wearing a sleeve during the day, and doing the exercises on their own."

COMBINED DECONGESTIVE THERAPY (CDT)

CDT combines MLD with bandaging, exercises, and skin care in the treatment of lymphedema. CDT can also involve breathing exercises and dietary instructions. CDT, like MLD, is becoming well known for the treatment of lymphedema and is taught in the training program at the Dr. Vodder School–North America.

CHAPTER 15

Craniosacral Therapy

Craniosacral therapy is a calming, subtle approach to bodywork that uses gentle touch to the head, neck, and back areas to relieve a variety of chronic pain patterns. In this modality, the craniosacral therapist's hands "listen" to the rhythm of the craniosacral system by touching the bones of the skull and spine. Through the process of manual listening, the therapist detects and gently corrects imbalances in the craniosacral system. Correcting and maintaining the balance of your craniosacral system can alleviate health problems ranging from TMJ to depression.

GETTING TO KNOW THE CRANIOSACRAL SYSTEM

Your health depends on the optimal functioning of this system. Yet, most people have never even heard of the craniosacral system. Learning a little bit about it can open your eyes to a new way of dealing with and preventing health problems that have not responded successfully to traditional treatment.

Where Is It?

The craniosacral system surrounds the brain and spinal cord, which comprise the central nervous system. The craniosacral system extends from the cranium (skull, head, and face) down to the sacrum (area of the tailbone), hence its name.

It is located underneath a flexible bony structure that includes the skull. Its membranes surround the brain, spinal cord, pituitary gland, and pineal glands.

What Is It?

The craniosacral system is one of the body's primary systems. It is composed of the network of meningeal membranes that surrounds the brain and spinal cord, the cerebrospinal fluid (CSF) that flows throughout these membranes, and the structures that pump the CSF throughout these membranes.

Cerebral spinal fluid is a clear, colorless liquid with a watery consistency. As it flows through the membranes surrounding the brain and spinal cord, the CSF carries vital nutrients that nourish the central nervous system. At the same time, the CSF and its surrounding membranes protect the brain and spinal cord from trauma and injury. The consistency of the CSF enables it to act as a shock absorber for the brain and protect it from the impact of blows from the environment. Cerebrospinal fluid is produced in the brain and is constantly reabsorbed and reformed throughout the day and night.

What Does the Craniosacral System Do?

The craniosacral system has an impact on the functioning of all the systems of the body and on the stability of emotions. It works optimally at a certain rhythm that helps maintain homeostasis, or balance, throughout the body and mind. The rhythm of the flow of cerebrospinal fluid throughout the membranes of this system is critical to its functioning.

Like other bodily fluids, such as blood and lymph, CSF circulates in a methodical sequence. The average person has approximately 125 milliliters (four ounces) of cerebrospinal fluid. It normally circulates within the membranes of the craniosacral system at a rate of six to twelve cycles every minute. If the rate were to slow down, due to trauma or systemic problems, the pumping of the CSF would become inefficient, and the system would eventually become sluggish. As a result, you could suffer from pain and discomfort, motor coordination problems, emotional problems, neurological dysfunctions, a loss of energy, and imbalances in other internal systems. You might also become more prone to illness.

KEEPING THE RHYTHM STEADY WITH CRANIOSACRAL THERAPY

In order to maintain harmony throughout the body's systems, the CSF needs to be pumped in a rhythmic fashion and at a consistent rate. That is where craniosacral therapy can help.

Goals of Treatment

The goal of this treatment is to affect the rhythm and flow of the cerebro-spinal fluid within these membranes. The CSF needs to flow smoothly so that it can nourish and balance the central nervous system. Encouraging the proper pumping and flow of CSF keeps the rhythm steady and optimal.

Establishing normal rhythm within the craniosacral system improves the functioning of the central nervous system (brain and spinal cord), which it surrounds. Keeping the brain and the nerves of the spinal cord humming smoothly is vital to the functioning of the whole mind-body system. Because the craniosacral system also surrounds and stimulates the pituitary and pineal glands, it has an enormous impact on the endocrine system, which controls our hormones, the chemical balance in our bodies, and our moods. Regulating the craniosacral system with craniosacral therapy paves the way for establishing homeostasis throughout the entire person.

Constrictions Are Released

It is through the gentle manipulation of the bony structure surrounding the craniosacral system that the therapist is able to correct and maintain the flow of CSF.

The craniosacral therapist gently manipulates the skull and bones around the sacrum to release contrictions in the membranes that surround the brain and spinal cord. It is the releasing of these constrictions that adjusts the rhythm of the movement of the cerebrospinal fluid. Balancing the flow of cerebrospinal fluid can bring relief from chronic pain not only in the head and jaw regions, which are touched directly, but throughout the entire body.

A Multitude of Benefits

Craniosacral therapy appears to correct underlying imbalances that maintain a wide array of problems that have not responded to traditional forms of treatment. Edward Feldman, a chiropractor in New Jersey who has incorporated craniosacral therapy into his practice, describes it as an exceedingly gentle modality that "lets the body respond to its own echo of what it is doing." Feldman further explains that by listening to the amplitude and fullness of the rhythm of the craniosacral system, the practitioner can get an idea of the vitality and health of the client. This makes craniosacral therapy a valuable assessment and prevention tool.

Feldman has found craniosacral therapy successful in alleviating chronic pain, headaches, TMJ (temporomandibular joint dysfunction), earaches, sinusitis, and asthma. He explains that the lack of transmission or blocked flow of CSF that contributes to these conditions can be corrected through the application of craniosacral therapy.

This form of therapy also addresses the fascia, the connective tissue that attaches to bones (via the muscle tendons) of the craniosacral system. Pain is often addressed in traditional medicine with medication, which can relieve symptoms but does not address the underlying cause of pain. Craniosacral therapy can alleviate the pain and discomfort caused when fascia in poor, rigid condition pulls on the muscles and bones beneath it. Unlike Rolfing (see chapter 17) or myofascial release, this modality uses a gentle approach to relax tight fascia.

In addition to correcting problems, balancing the rhythm of the craniosacral system fortifies your own internal healing mechanisms. Thus, as in the case of most bodywork modalities, craniosacral therapy is a preventive tool.

THE HISTORY OF CRANIOSACRAL THERAPY

Craniosacral therapy is designed to maintain your health, relieve chronic pain, and prevent future health problems by bringing about and stabilizing the optimal rate of pumping of the cerebrospinal fluid throughout the craniosacral system. This sounds simple enough. But first, you have to believe that the craniosacral system exists.

The existence of this critical system was not always accepted by the medical community. Even though a plausible case was made at the turn of the century by William G. Sutherland, an osteopathic physician, for the existence of the craniosacral system, his theories were not tested until the 1970s.

Sutherland believed, contrary to accepted "fact," that there are flexible points, or sutures, on the cranium. He proposed that the skull has to have the ability to move in a rhythmic fashion in response to hydraulic pressure caused by the pulsation of cerebrospinal fluid deep within the brain. Building on this concept, Sutherland used himself as a subject to see what would happen if the bones of his own skull were immobilized. The negative effects included depression and motor problems. He concluded that movement of the cranium is controlled by an internal system as critical as respiration. He published his findings in the late 1930s.

The medical profession was not ready at that time to consider a "new" internal system. The skull had always been viewed in traditional medicine as a static, unmoving structure whose sole function was to protect the brain from trauma and injury. The idea that the bones of the skull are flexible, that they could be easily manipulated, that the activity between the skull and the brain had a life of its own, and that this activity could be regulated challenged the deeply entrenched beliefs of the traditional medical community.

For generations, the medical profession remained skeptical about the existence of the craniosacral system. In the 1970s, it was proven not only to exist but also to have significant functions. At that time, a team of researchers led by John E. Upledger, an osteopath at the Osteopathic College of the University of Michigan, tested Sutherland's theories to determine whether there really is a craniosacral system and, if so, how it works.

Upledger's research demonstrated that there are micromovements in the cranium in response to movement in its surrounding membranes. This means that the skull is not a rigid structure, and significant activity lies just beneath it. His research further showed how to use the craniosacral system to assess a variety of health problems. Craniosacral therapists assess the strengths and weaknesses of an individual's state of health through the sense of touch. Considerable follow-up research has been performed on the craniosacral system as a separate bodily system that can be treated through manual manipulation of its bony covering.

Upledger's ongoing interest and research led to his development of craniosacral therapy for the treatment of imbalances in this vital system. In 1985, Upledger established the Upledger Institute in Palm Beach Gardens, Florida, as an educational resource and training center for craniosacral therapy. The practice and refinement of this modality have grown substantially due to Upledger's research and teaching. It has since been introduced to massage therapists, chiropractors, and physical therapists who incorporate it into their repertoire of healing practices. The Upledger Institute has trained more than twenty-seven thousand health care practitioners all over the world.

EXPERIENCING CRANIOSACRAL THERAPY

A session of craniosacral therapy lasts from forty-five to sixty minutes. The client remains fully clothed and seated in a comfortable posture in a padded chair. Only the areas of the head, face, neck, and spine are touched by the therapist. Craniosacral therapy allows you to correct problems physically removed from these areas without their having to be touched directly.

Be thorough when answering questions about your history. Even though craniosacral therapy is a safe and gentle modality, it is contraindicated in cases of recent stroke, cerebral aneurysm, and head injury. Consult your physician if you have any questions about receiving this form of bodywork.

The Assessment

Using highly skilled and sensitive touch, the therapist checks in all parts of the craniosacral system for restrictions that may be causing dysfunction and discomfort anywhere in the body.

The therapist feels with trained hands the rhythm of the movement of the cerebrospinal fluid. The rhythm consists of an amplitude and a number of cycles per minute. The fullness of the rhythm can also be felt and interpreted by the skilled, intuitive practitioner. Through this kinesthetic listening, the practitioner gets feedback and assesses the needs of the client. Sometimes the rate of expansion and contraction of the head is either slower or faster than it should be.

The Treatment

Once located by the feedback received through the therapist's hands, the restrictions are released through the gentle, rhythmic manipulation of the cranial bones of the skull, face, spinal column, sacrum, and coccyx (tailbone). The focus of the therapist is on the soft tissue, the muscles and fascia, surrounding the bones. Only the hands, no instruments, are used.

The therapist adjusts your craniosacral system with light but deliberate touches. The amount of pressure used to make corrections is very light. It takes only about 5 grams of pressure to allow the body to correct itself out of the pattern of distortion. The hands-on work is subtle and is designed to let the system unravel its own problems and correct itself.

Each separate release is achieved within seconds or minutes. As restrictions are released, the craniosacral system lets the rest of the body respond to the balancing of the rhythms in this key system. As a result, you may experience relief from long-standing pain. You may also experience a more steady, relaxed emotional state. However, it may take more than one session to correct imbalances.

THE BENEFITS OF CRANIOSACRAL THERAPY

Craniosacral therapy reestablishes normal rhythm within the craniosacral system. The benefits include improved functioning of the systems of the body, including the nervous, endocrine, and digestive systems.

This therapy can help relieve muscle tension and release pain. It can restore normal functioning if you experience chronic pain, recent injuries, headaches, facial pain, whiplash, jaw pain, chronic fatigue, nervousness, or immonosuppressive symptoms. Craniosacral therapy can alleviate earaches, sinusitis, and asthma.

Craniosacral therapy has emotional benefits as well. It has been shown to be effective in alleviating the symptoms of anxiety and depression. Recent work in craniosacral therapy has been done in the relief of "energy cysts,"

Benefits of Craniosacral Therapy

Restoration of normal rhythm within the craniosacral system.

Improved neural, hormonal, muscular, digestive, and brain functioning.

The body's state of health is assessed.

RELIEF FROM PROBLEMS CAUSED BY BLOCKAGES IN THE FLOW OF CSF:

* Chronic pain.

* Recent injuries.

* Headaches.

* Facial pain.

* Whiplash.

* Jaw pain and TMJ.

* Chronic fatigue.

* Nervousness.

* Earache.

* Sinusitis.

* Asthma.

* Depression.

* Anxiety.

* Attention deficit disorder.

* Autism.

* Brain injury.

constricted areas along the membranes of the system that hold emotional trauma. Through treatment with craniosacral therapy, victims of incest and other severe traumatic experiences have obtained relief by releasing muscle tension encapsulating the emotions and memories in the muscles of the craniosacral system.

Craniosacral therapy has also been shown to be effective in helping children. Parents who have gone the traditional route with limited results have obtained relief for their children in cases of attention deficit disorder, autism, and brain injuries.

Craniosacral therapy can be used as a preventive measure. Balancing the rhythm of this system helps maintain homeostasis and helps all the systems of the body, including the immune system, function more efficiently. Maintaining good health and fighting disease and pain depend on the vitality of your body's internal systems.

CHAPTER 16

The Rosen Method

The Rosen Method, developed by Marion Rosen, P.T., is a powerful modality distinguished by gentle touch that facilitates a process of self-discovery. Although the touch is relaxing, the Rosen Method is not massage. Rather, it is a form of bodywork in which the goal of the touch is to detect and make known to the receiver areas of holding. The holding takes the form of muscle tension that the receiver developed as a means of protection against experiencing painful feelings and memories.

According to Rosen, by cutting ourselves off from a part of ourselves, we also deprive ourselves of living fully. The Rosen Method gently guides individuals in the safe release of both the physical and emotional holding. The letting go of emotional and muscular barriers creates an opportunity for the blossoming of the person. Marion Rosen explains and demonstrates the relationships between our muscles and our emotions on an educational videotape available from the Rosen Center.

MUSCLES AND EMOTIONS

According to Rosen, musculature hardens as a physical defense against remembering experiences and feeling emotions that are difficult to face. Once the muscles tense and harden, they serve to hold the emotions down. The more reluctant we are to reveal to ourselves unpleasant experiences and emotions, the harder we hold the musculature. Some individuals tense their muscles to the point of chronic pain in an effort to obliterate the threatening feelings.

Out of Awareness

The feelings can be pushed down so far that they become subconscious, and, at that point, you no longer know you have them. If someone asked you about certain feelings, you might deny having them, not because you are being untruthful but because you have done such a good job of burying them. But they are there, lurking just under the surface, causing not only muscle pain but also a loss of receptivity to new experiences, a fear of taking emotional risks, and a narrow view of possibilities.

The effort put forth in holding the feelings and memories back is so enormous that you experience physical pain, become fatigued, and maintain an armor that deprives you of experiencing the love and caring offered by others. Rosen believes that 95 percent of back pain has its source in suppressed emotions.

The good news is that if you are willing to make the connection between your physical pain and your emotions, you can remember your feelings, feel them, and release yourself from their hold on you. Through the Rosen Method, the emotional discomfort is brief and the benefit is long-term.

A Point of Choice

The Rosen Method is designed to make you aware, in an environment of trust, of the stressed areas of your musculature. The awareness brings you to a point of choice. You can continue to hold back, hiding and allowing your fear to control you, or you can tackle your life and take risks even though you are afraid you will get hurt again. The touch and dialogue in the Rosen Method makes you aware of the options. Individuals will let go only when they are ready. Nothing is ever forced.

The cost of keeping the barriers intact is great because they shield you not only from the feelings you want to forget about but also from fully experiencing loving and caring feelings. On the other hand, the benefit of taking the barriers down is the reclaiming of your life. Individuals who have the courage to acknowledge the suppressed feelings can release themselves from the armor and lead more fulfilling lives. Everything you are becomes available to you. In addition to relief from muscular pain, you will have more energy, your life will be enriched by the loving feelings you allow in, and you will create the opportunity to reach your potential.

The positive changes are noticeable. Individuals who let go of their barriers look more relaxed in their faces and in their bodily movements. In some, the change can be considered a transformation.

Your Diaphragm Tells the Story

According to the theory of the Rosen Method, how your diaphragm moves as you breathe is a strong indicator of the extent to which your muscles are holding down your feelings. The diaphragm moves every time you breathe. How well the diaphragm moves has an impact on every aspect of your functioning.

When you breathe freely and without constriction, your diaphragm is supple and relaxed, moving up and down with ease. When the diaphragm moves freely and easily, it massages the internal organs and helps them function efficiently.

When your breathing is shallow, your diaphragm tightens up, causing all the nearby organs, including the heart, to work harder. Shallow breathing prevents sufficient oxygen from circulating throughout the systems of the body.

Rosen considers the diaphragm a muscle that picks up different feelings. She believes that everything that happens to you is played back to you in the way your diaphragm moves. The movement of the diaphragm is adversely affected when holding patterns persist. Observing and touching the diaphragm gives the Rosen Method practitioner information about your holding patterns.

THE HISTORY OF MARION ROSEN'S METHOD

Marion Rosen was born in Nuremberg, Germany, in 1914. When denied access to higher education in Nazi-era Germany, she persevered and studied privately with the leading professionals of the time in the practice of physical therapy and related treatments.

While still studying in Germany in the 1930s, Rosen worked with her mentor, Lucy Heyer, in the practice of relaxation techniques that focused on breathing, movement, and touch. They worked together with Gustav Heyer, Lucy's husband, a psychotherapist trained by Carl Jung. The three worked as a team. Rosen and her mentor prepared Gustav's patients before their psychotherapy sessions by inducing relaxation with breathing techniques and massage. The Rosen Method, developed years later, has its roots in Rosen's early career experiences, in which bodywork and relaxation were combined with verbal interaction to promote healing.

Because of the Nazi threat, Rosen was forced to flee her homeland for Sweden, where she studied physical therapy. She later emigrated to the United States, completed her physical therapy degree at the famous Mayo Clinic, and then settled in California, where she practiced physical therapy for many years.

In her physical therapy practice, Rosen noticed that as her clients' tight muscles softened, once-forgotten feelings and memories, both positive and negative, would sometimes come up. Over several decades, Rosen developed the theory that forgotten emotions and memories are stored in the body, causing constriction that leads to physical problems. This theory, based on her clinical observations, led naturally to the development of the Rosen Method.

By the mid-1970s, Rosen began to teach others how to use her method of touch combined with verbalization. In the early 1980s, the Rosen Institute, Berkeley, California, was established by a group of Rosen's students. It still sets the standards for training and provides instruction in the Rosen Method. To accommodate the growing demand for training, the Rosen Center East, Westport, Connecticut, was established in 1985. Certification training is intensive, requiring about four years to complete, including supervised sessions, personal sessions, and 350 client contact hours.

EXPERIENCING THE ROSEN METHOD

A Rosen Method session is about one hour in duration. This modality is done *with* the client, rather than *to* the client. As the client, you would lie under a blanket or sheet on a padded massage table in a quiet environment.

It is best to wear only underwear so that the practitioner can detect and touch directly the areas of holding. However, if you are more comfortable wearing additional clothing, you may. The practitioner will observe your breathing and the way you hold your body.

Type of Touch

In addition to careful observation, the Rosen Method practitioner makes physical contact with an open, sensitive hand and can feel if a muscle is contracted. The practitioner's hands are inquiring while touching, searching gently for hard areas that should be soft, and rigid areas that should move more freely. There is no application of force or strong pressure. There are no traditional massage strokes.

The type of touch used in the Rosen Method brings attention to the tautness, which represents the barrier between the client's buried emotions and the awareness and expression of those emotions. The touch is soft yet firm. The practitioner might hold his or her hand for a moment or two gently, but with its presence known, on a tight area, like the diaphragm or abdomen. The touch communication gradually facilitates the client's awareness and the process of letting go.

Touching and Talking

While touching an area that appears too hard or lacking in movement, the practitioner will ask questions designed to help you consider what you may be protecting or holding back. If you discussed a physical injury with the practitioner, he or she might ask you what was going on in your life at the time of the injury. According to Rosen, the emotions and life events at the time of the injury can contribute to the holding patterns. In the absence of injury, the practitioner might give you the feedback, while holding an open hand on your diaphragm, that this area does not show much movement as you breathe and ask you what you are holding back that is constricting your breathing. As the client, you can choose to share verbally as much or as little as you wish. You might even cry. The point is to make the connection within yourself between your emotions and your physical state.

The amount of time you feel uncomfortable with the newly uncovered emotion is short-lived. The predominant feeling is one of relief and freedom from pain. After the relief, you can experience a positive change and renewed energy.

The Rosen Method practitioner does not interpret, analyze, or judge what the client says or does. Rather, the practitioner in this modality is simply with the receiver, providing a supportive, welcoming environment. Rosen Method practitioners are trained in the art of presence and the skill of gentle touch. The goal of the practitioner is to be fully present in an accepting and nonintrusive way and to be respectful of whatever emerges during the session.

Individuals who engage in more than one session or who include the Rosen Method in their preventive health program find that more deeply entrenched and more subtle holdings can be released, producing further and ongoing personal growth.

THE BENEFITS OF THE ROSEN METHOD

The positive changes associated with the Rosen Method can affect you on many levels. Individuals receiving the Rosen Method experience themselves more fully and feel their aliveness. They have more energy because this precious resource is no longer being wasted on straining the muscles to hold down memories and emotions. When used in conjunction with psychotherapy, the Rosen Method can facilitate recovery from emotional trauma. The memories or emotions that are beneficial to release do not have to be old historically. A recent loss or disappointment could also have armature built around it. The Rosen Method gently helps release the feelings associated with both past and recent upsetting events.

Taking care of your inner life is considered by Rosen Method bodywork, and by all alternative health approaches, as a critical component of preventive health care. Thus, intertwined with the emotional benefits are the physical benefits. The following sequence demonstrates the reciprocal relationship between emotional and physical well-being:

1. The acknowledgment of holding back releases pent-up emotions and buried experiences.
2. The emotional awareness and subsequent release reduce muscle tension, which makes breathing less restricted.
3. Unrestricted breathing frees up the diaphragm, which massages and increases the efficiency of the internal organs attached to it and near it.
4. This positive rhythm spreads to all organs and systems of the entire body, producing efficient functioning and a harmonious internal environment.
5. When your body is functioning efficiently and harmoniously, your immune system can be more effective in preventing and fighting illness, and you feel even better emotionally.

WHEN THE ROSEN METHOD IS INDICATED
AND WHEN IT IS CONTRAINDICATED

The Rosen Method is primarily for emotionally stable individuals who want to become more in tune with themselves and flourish. It is not a replacement for psychotherapy.

The Rosen Method is not recommended for individuals suffering from a history of severe emotional disturbance or undergoing a current emotional crisis. Such individuals may not be ready for the release of their barriers and should be in the presence of trained mental health professionals for any process involving letting go of their defenses. If you suffer from an ongoing addiction or if you are on medication prescribed by a psychiatrist, be sure to inform the practitioner before embarking on the Rosen Method.

It is not designed to address acute physical pain or the chronic pain of severe illnesses. The pain best addressed by the Rosen Method is chronic muscle pain and tension—such as back pain and headaches—of emotional origin.

Benefits of the Rosen Method

Greater efficiency of internal organs and systems.

Greater awareness of inner feelings.

Progress in recovery from emotional trauma.

Gentle unblocking of muscular and emotional barriers.

Freer, less shallow breathing.

Relief from the symptoms of headaches, fatigue, and muscle tension.

More energy and vitality.

Greater freedom of movement.

Harmony between outer and inner self.

Individuals are better able to reach their potential.

Learning How to Integrate and Move Your Body

Rolfing

Hellerwork

The Alexander Technique

The Feldenkrais Method

Each of the modalities included in this section addresses in its own way the structure of the body as a whole and how its parts fit and move together. Each requires a commitment from the receiver to work toward achieving his or her personal goals, with the help of the practitioner. Undergoing bodywork that addresses the integration of the person can lead to significant and lasting change.

CHAPTER 17

Rolfing

Rolfing is an established method of body-work that was created and developed by Ida P. Rolf, who earned her doctorate in biophysics in the 1920s. Motivated by her desire to overcome a family illness, Rolf sought solutions outside the boundaries of traditional medicine. She began her work in the 1930s, but it was not until the 1960s that she taught her methods to others. She named the modality that she developed *structural integration.* Her students, who respected her enormously as a researcher, practitioner, and teacher, called this form of bodywork Rolfing.

Today, Rolfing is considered a mind-body system within the larger framework of structural integration. It is a system of deep muscular manipulation and movement education that corrects the effects that time, trauma, and injury have had on the body.

The goal of Rolfing is to release the rigidity and tightness of the body's soft tissue through the processes of deep tissue massage and bodywork so that the body can become more flexible and achieve a healthier alignment. Rolfing goes beyond the modalities that help relieve chronic tension and pain because of its focus on renewing and revitalizing the structure of the body as a whole. Rolfing differs from all other modalities in that it uses the force of gravity as a tool. It is a powerful approach with a positive impact on physical and emotional functioning that can last a lifetime.

A HOLISTIC APPROACH

Rolfing is a holistic form of bodywork. In this modality, the parts of the body are viewed and treated as interrelated units that form a whole that is greater than the sum of its parts. Rolf considered her structural integration system a form of treatment aimed at the integration of the whole person. During her career, Rolf worked with Fritz Perls, the psychologist who founded Gestalt psychotherapy, a school of therapy based on holistic principles in the field of mental health. In fact, the foundation of Rolfing is a creative integration of mind-body processes.

The term *integration* is key to understanding the essence of Rolfing as a holistic modality. On one level, integration refers to realigning the parts of the body such that they move away from the distorted, poorly integrated, misshapen form they have become and go back to their original, healthy, integrated relationship with each other.

What caused the healthy integration to fall apart? It is a gradual, insidious process due to the effects of gravity, the imitation of the poor posture of role models, and other physical and emotional factors. Of all possible factors, gravity is considered in Rolfing as the main reason the body becomes misaligned.

On an even deeper level, Rolfing is designed to integrate the whole person by bringing into focus the interrelationships among body, mind, emotions, and our everyday environment. With increased flexibility and better body alignment come increased vitality, clarity of thought, and a release of blockages in emotional feeling and expression.

THE BODY'S MISALIGNMENT

The misalignment of the body occurs gradually and subtly. It is caused over a long period of time by the pull of gravity and by physical stress reactions to life experiences. Misalignment is reflected in bodily posture. The goal of Rolfing is to realign the body in such a way as to let gravity flow through it. As you can see in Figures 17.1 and 17.2, the body is visibly different in its misaligned and realigned states.

The Role of Gravity in Misalignment

According to Rolf, from the time we are born we are subjected to forces and life experiences that take our bodies out of healthy alignment. Over time, our body parts change their position in relationship to each other, and our bodies become misshapen. The main culprit is gravity, an inescapable negative force on body alignment. From the time we learn to stand upright, our body's posture becomes susceptible to the downward pull of gravity. Examples of the effects of gravity and other culprits include one shoulder held higher than the other, a protruding neck and chin, or a slumped posture. Aside from these more obvious structural problems, gravity can also contribute to feelings of chronic fatigue and sluggishness. The process of misalignment occurs so gradually that you would not necessarily notice that it was happening.

The Impact of Misalignment on the Fascia

As the process of misalignment progresses, the fascia throughout the body becomes increasingly distorted and rigid. Fascia is a complex web of interwoven, interconnected tissue found throughout the entire structure of the body. It is the soft tissue that surrounds and holds the muscles, organs, and bones of the body. The release and the health of the fascia is the focus of myofascial release therapy described in chapter 9.

In Rolfing, fascia is viewed as a system of support because it gives the body shape. When the fascia is healthy and flexible, the body moves freely and without discomfort. As the body moves further out of alignment, the fascia loses its suppleness. As the misaligned postures begin to take hold, the dysfunctional postures begin to feel natural. The fascia fixes itself around the misaligned structure and becomes part of it. When the fascia rigidifies in this way, it holds on too tightly to the muscles, organs, and bones, causing imbalances in bodily systems, increasingly poor posture, and chronic pain.

Although the existence of fascia was known for a long time before Rolfing was developed, the significance of fascia in our daily functioning and health had been underestimated. The role and significance of fascia are still ignored by most of the traditional medical community. Rolf believed that if the fascia were examined and properly treated by traditional medical doctors, pain relief would be available to more people.

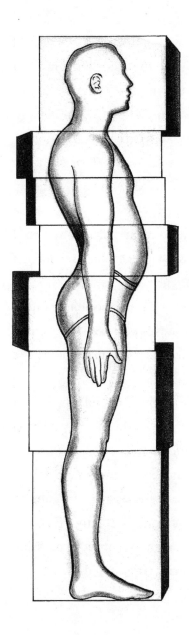

Figure 17.1   Body Misalignment

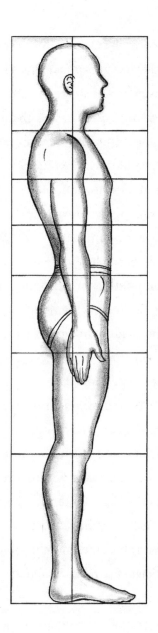

Figure 17.2   Lining up the Body

Emotional Consequences of Misalignment

In addition to experiencing physical distress due to the rigidity and tension in fascial tissue, there are also emotional consequences to bodily misalignment. An aspect of the theory underlying Rolfing is that as your body becomes inflexible, the spontaneous experience and expression of emotion become blocked. Throughout the course of development, all of us suffer some degree of emotional trauma. When we do, we react with bodily tension and misaligned movements.

For example, think about how a child who is being yelled at by a parent, embarrassed by a teacher, or teased by a group of peers on a school bus might hold his or her body during such experiences. In the theory underlying Rolfing, your emotional traumas, both big and small, become trapped in the rigidified body structure. As your body moves out of a state of natural alignment and into a condition of inflexibility, your emotional range can become limited.

Your emotional tone can become progressively more dulled over the years as your body's musculature becomes rigidly held in a misaligned position. Your emotional responses to situations and to other people can become automatic habitual responses rather than spontaneous reactions.

Rolfing counteracts the forces that have caused bodily misalignment and makes the body receptive to returning to its original, healthy shape. As the body becomes more flexible and the misalignment is reduced, emotional blockages are released and vitality and spontaneity are restored.

THE BODY AS A PLASTIC MEDIUM

The fascia, which is supposed to move easily and allow for freedom of motion, can become traumatized and frozen through injury, bad postural habits, and gravity. Rolf considers gravity the main culprit behind the body's misalignment.

Fortunately, fascia is a flexible, pliable web of tissue. Because of this important fact, the body is capable of being realigned no matter how mis-aligned and rigid it may have become. The fascia, through the Rolfing process, can be manipulated in such a fashion as to remold the shape of the entire body. The Rolfing process is designed to correct misalignment so that posture, flexibility, and range of motion are improved, and the body is restored to the way it was before gravity and life experiences distorted it. It is this concept—that the body is a plastic medium—that is the hallmark of the Rolfing process.

ROLFING VERSUS MYOFASCIAL RELEASE

Like myofascial release, Rolfing involves deep-tissue work and relieves chronic pain by releasing the fascia, the tissue that surrounds and connects the muscles. However, in the myofascial release modality, the release of the fascia is performed mostly for the purposes of pain reduction and increased range of motion. In Rolfing, an added dimension and the main focus is the correction and enhancement of the body's structural integration.

Thus, in addition to working on deep tissue to relieve chronic pain, Rolfing uses the body's plasticity to bring its major segments (head, shoul-der, thorax, pelvis, and legs) into a finer vertical alignment. The goal of alignment is to establish the horizontality of the pelvis. The alignment of the pelvis is also a guiding principle in myofascial release therapy. However, alignment of the pelvis is not planned in myofascial release therapy as a spe-cific step on the way to completing a predetermined sequence of sessions as it is in Rolfing.

THE ROLFING EXPERIENCE AND
THE REALIGNMENT OF THE BODY

As part of the assessment of structural problems and progress, Rolfers take pictures of their clients from all angles before and after treatment. These pictures serve two purposes: They provide feedback to both the practitioner and the client on the body's alignment before the hands-on work begins, and they show visible changes in the body's alignment after bodywork is performed.

The client wears underwear, and no oil is used. The purpose of using no oil is to maximize the friction so that the fascia will move out of a rigid state. As the client, you would lie flat on a bodywork table as the Rolfer pushes and slides across the surface of your skin.

Is Rolfing Painful?

In order to move the fascia out of its rigid state, the Rolfer has to exert sufficient pressure to stretch this tissue. Does this process cause pain?

According to Caroline May, an advanced certified Rolfer who was mentored by Ida Rolf, "The degree of discomfort or pain experienced depends mostly on your own personal perception of pain." She explained that some of her clients will flinch at the slightest touch on a rigid area, whereas others insist that deep pressure feels good and is never painful.

For most people, although the release of rigid fascia can cause feelings of momentary discomfort or pain, the pain is usually fleeting. It often disappears as soon as pressure is removed and is not the primary experience of Rolfing. That Rolfing can be performed gently is evidenced by its use on infants and senior citizens.

According to May, the majority of individuals who experience Rolfing report pleasure derived from firm massage and release of tension. As the fascia is freed and the muscles begin to relax, many clients report a feeling of lightness and well-being.

Rolfing and Emotional Release

Sometimes, clients experience emotional release along with the release of muscular tension. Often, the revival of past emotional experiences is elicited by the bodywork on those parts of the body that were affected by the original experience. Rolfers are trained to help you in a sensitive way with the emotions you may feel and wish to express as muscular tension is released. The combination of physical and emotional release can produce a strong sense of well-being.

The Rolfing Series

Although you can choose to engage in one Rolfing session at a time at your discretion, Rolfing usually takes place over a series of ten organized sessions, moving from part to whole, from superficial to deep, according to a logical scheme aimed at the realignment of the body. By the end of the series, your body is brought into harmony with gravity. Each session lasts from sixty to ninety minutes.

The Early Sessions

The first three Rolfing sessions work on the release of the superficial fascia—the outermost layer of fascia, just beneath the surface of the skin. As the superficial fascia stretches and detaches from the muscle and bone, deeper structures are freed and begin to reorganize themselves.

This superficial layer of fascia is referred to by Rolfers as the body's stocking. The stocking must be freed before further work can be done. Most clients feel relief after the very first session, because the freeing of the fascia surrounding the rib cage helps them breath more freely, which in turn supplies the brain with more oxygen and gives them more energy. Ease of movement is also experienced by many clients after the stocking is freed.

The focus of the second session is on the legs and feet, those parts of the body that connect us with the earth. The purpose of the session is to help the legs and feet support the weight of the body in a more centered manner, making standing and walking less of an effort. Most clients notice a difference between the Rolfed leg and the not-yet-Rolfed leg when asked to walk around in the middle of the session before the second leg is worked on. Work is also done on the back and neck during the second session.

The purpose of the third Rolfing session is to integrate the work performed in the first two sessions. During the third session, the shoulders, ribs, and pelvis are arranged into an even stack, resulting in freer breathing and less crowding of the structures. The end of the third session is considered a critical point in treatment. At this point, the client has the option of a longer waiting period before proceeding to the next phase of treatment, which focuses on the core of the body.

The Body-Core Sessions

Sessions four through seven focus on the active core of the body. This consists of deeper layers of fascia and the parts of the body closest to the spine and the midline of the body. The goal of the fourth sessions is to improve the support of the structures that compose the pelvic floor. Remember that the goal of realignment is to reestablish the horizontality of the pelvis, thus making this central structure stand in harmony with gravity.

By the seventh session, the pelvis has been placed in the proper horizontal position. Also during the seventh session, the Rolfer helps to further improve your breathing by releasing the fascia of the neck, skull, and face that constrict the nasal passages. Many clients have reported the easing of emotional distress by the end of the body-core sessions.

The Integrative Sessions

Whereas the first seven sessions concentrated on different parts of the body, the last three sessions focus on the body as a whole unit and integrate the bodywork that has been done. The bodywork in these last session deals with movement of the body as a whole in relation to gravity. The client is taught to use gravity, allowing the gravity to flow through the body, rather than allowing gravity to work against the body. Through this educational process, you learn how to use your new body and maintain its realignment.

Advanced Rolfing

Refresher sessions are offered six months to one year after the completion of the Rolfing series. The purpose of these sessions is to help you maintain your gains. The advanced sequence focuses on balanced movement in the face of gravity.

THE BENEFITS OF ROLFING

We all experience the impact of misalignment in different ways, which may include slumped posture, muscular aches and pains, and emotional weariness, all of which contribute to physical and mental stress. Fortunately, through Rolfing, these problems are reversible. The body can be restored to its natural, original shape. Once the natural shape of your body is restored and maintained, you experience an increase in physical and emotional well-being. The realignment helps fight against the visible aspects of the aging process, including slumped posture and sagging muscles.

Other benefits of Rolfing include the more efficient use of the muscles, more economical and graceful bodily movement, increased energy, and a reduction in chronic physical and mental stress. The improvement in the use of your muscles provides relief from the pain associated with poor posture, an increase in your flexibility and range of motion, better coordination, and less stiffness. Rolfing also results in increased physiological efficiency, because it improves your breathing, circulation, digestion, elimination, and sleep patterns.

The benefits of Rolfing take place on more than one level. On the surface, Rolfing can improve your appearance, because how you hold your body, your posture, your body shape, and your comfort in your body all affect how you look to yourself and others. On another level, Rolfing increases the suppleness of the muscles, allowing you to move with greater freedom. On an emotional level, Rolfing allows for the release of negative emotions and the emergence of feelings of well-being.

WHO SHOULD NOT UNDERGO ROLFING?

Because of the amount of physical pressure involved in the Rolfing process, it is recommended that individuals suffering with acute pain, illness, or prolonged, major addiction should not undergo Rolfing. Rolfing should also be avoided if you have a fever, are suffering from vomiting, nausea, diarrhea, pain of unknown origin, arthritis, jaundice, cancer, bleeding, acute phlebitis, thrombosis, varicose veins, high blood pressure, or heart problems. If you are pregnant, consult your physician before receiving bodywork.

THE ROLF INSTITUTE

The Rolf Institute in Boulder, Colorado, was founded in 1971 by Ida Rolf. This organization is the official training institution for Rolfing practitioners. More that nine hundred Rolfers, who practice internationally, have been trained and certified by the Rolf Institute's vigorous program. Rolfing is practiced in more than twenty nations. The Rolf Institute, which has offices in Germany and Brazil as well as in the United States, supports research on structural integration and promotes Rolfing to the public all over the world.

Benefits of Rolfing

Alignment of the body as an integrated whole.

Improved posture, appearance, ease of movement, and coordination.

Fewer muscular aches and pains and less stiffness.

Greater flexibility and range of motion.

Improved suppleness of muscle tissue.

Increased body awareness.

Diminished signs of aging, e.g., slumped posture and sagging muscles.

Improved breathing, circulation, digestion, elimination, and sleep patterns.

Release of long-held negative emotions, resulting in increased feelings of well-being.

Better stress management and coping.

Enhanced personal growth.

CHAPTER 18

Hellerwork

Hellerwork, founded by Joseph Heller in 1978, is an integrated system of bodywork that combines deep-tissue work, a movement reeducation process, and therapeutic dialogue. These components of Hellerwork interact to restore the body, as a whole, to its original condition. Although Hellerwork was inspired by Rolfing and is based on many of the same principles, the bodywork system designed by Heller makes this modality unique.

Hellerwork is given in a set series of sessions that allows the restoration of the body to unfold in a logical sequence. Undergoing Hellerwork can free you from the physical and mental components of stress. Incorporating the fundamental principles of Hellerwork into your everyday life can make the gains long-lasting.

A MODALITY FOR PERSONAL GROWTH

Hellerwork is not considered a remedy for illness; rather, it is a process designed to enhance personal growth. When you participate in Hellerwork, you are moved from your current state to a more optimal state of health and well-being. This optimal state of health is considered in Hellerwork theory to be the body's normal, original, natural condition. Thus, the focus of Hellerwork is to return the body to a more aligned, relaxed, and youthful state, the way it was before it was adversely affected by the ravages of gravity and negative emotions.

Change and growth on deeper levels are triggered by the physical changes. Thus, this form of bodywork enhances the restoration and blossoming of the whole person.

A fundamental premise of Hellerwork is that no matter how much bodywork a person receives, poor postures and old movement patterns will gradually return unless the person is armed with information and techniques for maintaining and building on the gains. Once the physical gains diminish, emotions can become blocked again, and personal growth can slow down or stop. It is for this reason that movement education and therapeutic dialogue are included in this modality.

The movement education helps you more naturally perform everyday movements such as standing, bending, walking, sitting, and reaching. When you move with better bodily alignment and less strain, tension is diminished and energy is enhanced.

As the body is restored, the inner self journeys through a healing process as well. This process is guided gently and sensitively by the Hellerwork practitioner, who talks with the receiver about memories and emotions that come up during the sessions. Verbal expression on the part of the receiver is encouraged by the Hellerwork practitioner, who facilitates the receiver's making connections between the bodily sensations and underlying thoughts and emotions. It is through making these connections that change can be profound and long-lasting.

JOSEPH HELLER AND THE HISTORY OF HELLERWORK

Joseph Heller was born in Poland in 1940. To escape from the threat of Nazism, Heller emigrated to Russia, and then to Paris. He settled in Los Angeles in 1957, at age seventeen, and has remained in the United States since then. Before he developed his interest in bodywork, Heller was an aerospace engineer.

After experiencing Rolfing as a client, he was so impressed with its positive impact that he decided to become a bodywork practitioner. Heller's training as an engineer influenced the way he conceptualized the structure and movement of the human body. He was trained by Ida Rolf and became a Rolfer in 1972. In addition to studying with Rolf, Heller also studied with Judith Aston, an expert in the patterns of body movement.

In 1975, Heller became the first president of the Rolf Institute. It was not long before he became internationally known as a somatic educator, one who teaches the proper use of the body. By 1978, Heller developed his own modality, known as Hellerwork, in which he combined: (1) the concepts of deep-tissue work and alignment of Rolfing; (2) the principles of bodily movement developed by Judith Aston; (3) the verbal release of emotions he noticed when he gave bodywork; and (4) the conceptualization of the human body as an integrated system, based on Heller's engineering background.

Heller has trained hundreds of practitioners around the world in Hellerwork. Only certified Hellerwork practitioners can practice this modality. Practitioners are certified by Hellerwork International, which maintains high professional standards and is responsible for the continuing education of Hellerwork practitioners.

MASSAGE, MOVEMENT, AND THE MIND

There are three elements of Hellerwork that are present in each session. These elements are intertwined to form a cohesive, integrated program.

Massage

The massage element of Hellerwork consists of deep-tissue bodywork to relieve tension in your connective tissue, or fascia, by stretching it back to its normal position, so the body can return to its natural alignment. Fascia is a pliable tissue that is interwoven throughout the body and wraps around the muscles and bones to form a multilayered body stocking.

Fascia in a healthy condition is loose, flexible, and moist. When the fascia becomes rigid and adheres too tightly to bone and muscle, the alignment of the body becomes distorted and out of balance. Tight and rigid fascia contributes to physical tension and stress. A more complete description of the characteristics of fascia and the role it plays in our everyday functioning is provided in chapter 9 on myofascial release therapy and in chapter 17 on Rolfing.

The focus of the massage component of Hellerwork is on releasing tight, rigidified fascia. This level of tissue release requires deep-tissue massage. This deep work results in profound relief of tension and stress. The loosening up of the body allows it to move more freely and naturally.

Movement Reeducation

Freer movement in Hellerwork is not simply a by-product of the massage. Rather, movement is assessed, worked on, and practiced in its own right. Hellerwork includes a process of movement reeducation, in which video feedback helps the client more effectively perform such everyday movements as standing, sitting, walking, bending, and reaching. Movement of the body as a whole is integrated toward the end of the sequence.

The Mind

According to Heller, thoughts and feelings are held in the body. Hellerwork includes verbal dialogue that allows you to see the relationship between your emotions and your body—i.e., how you hold emotions in your body and how to release particular emotions that are held in particular body parts.

The therapeutic discussion between practitioner and client is related to the particular part of the body that is the focus of that session. For example, the dialogue during the session on feet and legs would center around issues of groundedness and standing on your own two feet, whereas dialogue during the session on the back would center on the holding back and releasing of emotions. The purpose of including this component is to enhance personal growth, which is achieved by encouraging release on a deeper level. Revealing emotions is never forced; it is gently encouraged.

THE HELLERWORK SEQUENCE

Generally, Hellerwork consists of eleven sessions, each lasting ninety minutes and focusing on a different part of the body in a prearranged sequence. As the sessions progress, the client moves from superficial to deeper levels of resolving body-mind-movement issues.

Each session of Hellerwork contains elements of the three Ms—massage, movement, and the mind. Each session focuses on a different part of the body, each with its own significance to deeper levels of functioning. The focus and theme of each session are summarized in Table 18.1.

A Developmental Sequence

The series of eleven sessions in Table 18.1 is organized according to the sequence of human development. The early sessions on breathing, standing up, and reaching out (1, 2, and 3) address the issues of infancy and early childhood. The middle, or core, sessions on control and surrender, gut feelings, holding back feelings, and intellect (4, 5, 6, and 7) address the issues of adolescence. The last four sessions in the Hellerwork sequence (8, 9, 10, and 11) integrate all levels of the person, making the person ready to face the world with greater vitality and self-knowledge.

It All Starts with Breathing

Notice that the first session in the Hellerwork sequence focuses on breathing. Breathing is equated in Hellerwork with inspiration. *The Hellerwork Client Handbook* explains that the way you breathe affects your energy level, your feelings of vitality, and your ability to fulfill your potential as a person. Breathing can be made easier and fuller by releasing muscles surrounding the rib cage and chest, by sitting and standing properly, and by mentally connecting your breathing patterns to your emotions.

Learning to breathe properly takes practice. Poor breathing is in part a bad habit that can be changed. Change requires paying attention and focusing on your breathing patterns. You can notice changes in your breathing as you move and as you experience emotions. When you are tense, your

TABLE 18.1   THE HELLERWORK SEQUENCE

Session		Parts of Body	Theme
1	Inspiration	Rib cage and surrounding muscles	Open up breathing to increase life energy and to feel inspired
2	Standing on Your Own Two Feet	Feet and legs	Alignment with earth for self-support and sufficiency
3	Reaching Out	Arms, shoulders, torso	Giving and receiving; assertiveness
4	Control and Surrender	Core: inner torso; inner thighs	Learning how to release
5	The Guts	Stomach muscles	Gut feelings
6	Holding Back	Spine and back muscles	Holding back feelings
7	Losing Your Head	Face, head, neck	Alignment of head over torso; the mind-body connection
8	The Feminine	Legs, feet, pelvis	Expression of feminine energy
9	The Masculine	Arms, shoulders, rib cage, neck	Expression of masculine energy
10	Integration	Major joints: ankles, knees, hips, shoulders, elbows, wrists, spine	Integration of the whole person
11	Coming Out	The inner self	Full self-expression

breathing can become shallow. You might not even breathe at all for a short time. The oxygen deprivation created by shallow breathing can make you feel light-headed and prevent you from thinking clearly, thereby adding to your stress. Giving yourself the message to breathe fully during those tense moments can bring relief.

EXPERIENCING HELLERWORK

Hellerwork is an educational bodywork and movement program that consists of the eleven sessions described in Table 18.1. In the first session, the practitioner will explain the nature of Hellerwork and what to expect. The practitioner will also take a history and ask you about your goals in undertaking this form of bodywork.

As the client, you are asked to disrobe to your underwear or minimal clothing. Videos are often taken of the client walking and sitting in order to provide before-and-after feedback. The bodywork is performed on a padded bodywork table.

Each session is about ninety minutes, with approximately sixty minutes of bodywork and the remainder devoted to movement education and therapeutic dialogue, which are intertwined with the bodywork component. For example, the practitioner might ask you to get off the table and walk around after releasing the connective tissue in the first leg, before the other leg is worked on. Walking at this point will allow you to feel the difference. Feeling the difference while you are in motion provides your brain with valuable feedback, which will enhance your gains.

When the practitioner encounters tight areas of your fascia, he or she might provide you with images that help you release. The practitioner might ask you what you are feeling or thinking, to give you the opportunity for free self-expression.

As you progress through the sessions, you will become more accustomed to the interplay of bodywork, movement, and dialogue. You will experience positive changes in your physical, mental, and emotional functioning.

After you complete the sequence, your body will be in a state of balance and healthy alignment. You can maintain and enhance that state if you continue to practice the movement education provided as part of Hellerwork. Follow-up sessions are available for maintaining gains and for bringing your body back into alignment if you undergo physical or emotional trauma in the future.

LOSING YOUR HEAD: VALERIE'S EXPERIENCE

In 1987, I experienced Hellerwork—the full series—as a favor to my massage therapist, Debra, who was planning to move to California after earning her certification in this modality. She needed a volunteer to undergo Hellerwork with a certified practitioner as she watched and participated as an apprentice. She thought that, as a psychologist, I would be intrigued by the interweaving of body, mind, and emotions that is central to Hellerwork. Debra was right. I decided to go on this adventure.

At the first session, the Hellerwork practitioner, Susan, asked thought-provoking questions in a gentle manner as she recorded my responses on a form. She wanted to know why I volunteered and what I hoped to gain personally from the process. She asked me about my commitment to my well-being.

It was during the intake that I discovered that I did not include my head as a part of my body. I described my body as everything from the neck down. I saw my head as my brain rather than as a body part that housed my brain. I was astonished and somewhat embarrassed about the implications of my perception of myself. Susan looked at me as though she was not surprised. She explained that the detachment of mind and body was not unusual, particularly for people who think a lot. We made mind-body integration one of the goals in my Hellerwork program.

Every session of Hellerwork was powerful and positive for me. I looked forward to each meeting with Susan with a sense of adventure. I remember my eagerness as we approached Session 7: Losing Your Head.

The goals of the Losing Your Head session included the alignment of the head over the torso and the enhancement of the mind-body connection. For me, the greatest value of the session, and of Hellerwork in general, was a reorientation of my perception of my body, from a vehicle used for carrying my head around to an integrated whole that works together with my mind and emotions.

As was the case in all sessions, Losing Your Head included bodywork, verbal interaction, and movement. The bodywork consisted of loosening the muscles and fascia in the head, neck, and upper back with deep-tissue massage. In addition to approaching these body parts as I lay on my stomach, Susan also had me turn over so that she could reach underneath and use the weight of my body to facilitate the process.

When she encountered resistance in the fascia, Susan would ask me to visualize the area "melting like butter" as I felt the warmth emanating from her fingers. I was delighted to experience my body respond so readily to my mental images. As I lay on my back, she held my head gently in her two hands. She instructed me to let it go, stating with good humor, "Don't worry, I won't let it fall off." I gave in immediately, trusting my head to stay intact without strain.

In addition to the bodywork, verbal suggestions, and mental imagery, Susan asked me to get up and walk around, allowing my head to stay up and centered on its own. I could feel it balancing naturally on top of the rest of my body. I did not have to work to hold it in place. I felt good as I walked around the room, experiencing my head as integrated with the rest of my body. I could actually sense a closer relationship evolving between my body, my mind, and my emotions.

My Hellerwork experience enhanced both my personal life and my work as a psychologist. It was a turning point that led to my being more in tune with myself and more authentic with others.

THE BENEFITS OF HELLERWORK

The benefits of Hellerwork take place on many levels. The bottom line is the enhancement of personal growth. In Hellerwork, the growth of the inner person is achieved through balancing and integrating the body. Improvement in posture, increased grace and flexibility, and more efficient movement patterns help you feel better physically, mentally, emotionally, and spiritually. Hellerwork helps you make connections between your inner life and your physical being, thereby increasing self-awareness. Improving your relationship with yourself enhances your relationships with others and your adaptation to the inevitable changes over the course of a lifetime.

The restoration of the body achieved through Hellerwork helps eliminate chronic pain, increases your energy and creativity, and helps you maintain your youthful vitality and ease of movement as you age. Moving with fluidity as you get older helps you maintain flexibility in your attitudes and relationships.

Benefits of Hellerwork

Restoration of the body to its original, natural state.

Enhanced physical, mental, emotional, and spiritual well-being.

Enhanced personal growth.

A more balanced and integrated body.

Better posture.

More grace and flexibility.

More efficient movement patterns.

An understanding of the connections between your inner life and your physical being.

Heightened self-awareness.

A better relationship with yourself.

Better relationships with others.

Easier adaptation to the inevitable changes that occur over the course of a lifetime.

Elimination of chronic pain.

Increased energy and creativity.

Greater ability to maintain youthful vitality and ease of movement as you age.

Greater ability to maintain flexibility in your attitudes and relationships as you age.

CHAPTER 19

The Alexander Technique

The Alexander Technique was developed by Frederick Matthias Alexander at the beginning of the twentieth century. It is one of the oldest forms of Western bodywork still in use today. The goal of this modality is to help you better use your body. Proper use of the body facilitates ease and freedom of movement, lengthens the spine, supports your head on your neck without strain, and promotes coordination in the performance of everyday activities. Improper use of the body results in strained muscles and feeling stressed and fatigued.

The Alexander Technique was designed as an educational process. It is a form of mind-body education based on the premise that positive changes in alignment and breathing can lead to positive life changes. Many singers and other performers have learned through the Alexander Technique to make their bodies move in such a way as to achieve their goals. Even if you are not a performer, learning how to use your body more effectively can relieve muscle tension, improve your posture, boost your self-confidence, and enhance your vitality. You can learn how to do tasks as varied as working at a computer, lifting young children, or talking in front of a group with greater ease and less muscle strain.

THE HISTORY OF ALEXANDER LESSONS

Frederick Matthias Alexander, born in 1869, was an Australian Shakespearean actor who delivered dramatic monologues in front of live audiences. Shortly into his career, he developed vocal problems and suffered from fatigue. Difficulty projecting his voice and losing his voice during performances threatened his career.

When numerous doctors were unable to help him, Alexander decided to find a solution on his own. He suspected intuitively that the crux of the problem resided in his posture and bodily movement, particularly the positioning of the head and neck areas. By devising a system of mirrors placed at various angles, he observed himself as he stood and spoke.

Beginning in 1890, Alexander devoted the next ten years to examining and correcting how he used his body. He made detailed self-observations, noting postural positions that made him lose his voice. He took corrective actions that created better balance in the relationship of head to neck to spine. The postural and movement corrections he made helped his voice return to normal.

After reeducating himself on how to use his body more effectively, he wanted to share his technique with others. Performers who wanted to improve how they came across to the audience became interested in learning what Alexander knew. It was not long before he began to formalize his bodywork in what became known as the Alexander Technique.

The Alexander Technique was taught through a course of individualized instruction known as Alexander Lessons. These lessons were designed to organize the teaching and learning of the technique to suit the needs and goals of each individual.

By the early 1900s, Alexander Lessons were fashionable. Alexander moved from Australia to Western Europe to spread the word about his effective methods for correcting postural and vocal problems. The Alexander Technique was taught to actors, singers, teachers, musicians, and others who wanted to improve the way they moved and used their bodies. It was not long before Alexander's work spread throughout the world.

After World War II, the growth of this modality was interrupted because so many of Alexander's students were killed in action. In the 1960s, a resurgence of interest in this form of bodywork led to the opening in New York City of the American Center for the Alexander Technique, the first center in the United States to offer training in the Alexander Technique. In recent years, his techniques have been used at major educational institutions, including New York University, the Julliard School, Boston University, the London Academy of Music and Dramatic Art, and England's New College of Speech and Drama.

In 1987, the North American Society of Teachers of the Alexander Technique (NASTAT) was established to maintain the high standards set by the original society established in London. NASTAT trains and certifies teachers of the Alexander Technique in the United States and is highly selective before accepting applicants into its rigorous training and certification program. Approximately half of the three hundred teachers of the Alexander

Technique in the United States received training at the American Center for the Alexander Technique in New York City.

THE THEORY UNDERLYING THE ALEXANDER TECHNIQUE

The theory underlying the Alexander Technique is that learning to use your body more effectively can alleviate a variety of posture and movement-related problems. Continuing to move your body incorrectly may be at the root of muscle pain and respiratory difficulties.

How You Learn to Misuse Your Body

The misuse of the body is a learned process that starts at an early age. The body moves into a state of misalignment as it tries to adapt to such stresses as being handled improperly in infancy and early childhood, emotional and physical trauma, and being forced to sit in uncomfortable chairs in school.

Through conditioning, the misalignment becomes habitual and automatic. As adults, we continue to compensate for the misalignment that developed in the early years of life. This compensation can throw the entire body out of alignment. Through the unrelenting misuse of our bodies, we cause ourselves to suffer from chronic physical problems, stress, and tension.

The Consequences of Misusing Your Body

The continual misuse of the body creates and maintains a variety of physical problems that become chronic and interfere with accomplishing the tasks of everyday life. Moving inefficiently and incorrectly strains the muscles and is an energy drain.

The recurring physical problems associated with incorrect posture and movement patterns include:

- ❧ Chronic back pain.
- ❧ Chronic neck and shoulder pain.
- ❧ Restricted breathing patterns.
- ❧ Poor voice projection.
- ❧ Loss of voice while speaking or singing.
- ❧ Constant low energy and exhaustion.
- ❧ Unexplained limitations in performing a task or sport.

The misuse of the body can contribute to internal problems as well. If your posture is slumped or otherwise distorted, your musculature will become compressed and contracted. In addition to causing you physical pain, the poor postural habits put excess pressure on your internal organs and restrict the space around them, thereby making them work harder and less efficiently. Such systems as respiration, digestion, and elimination are adversely affected by poor posture and muscle strain. These vital functions are supported through an improvement in overall posture.

Alexander theorized and demonstrated that alleviating such problems requires correcting the misalignment. The Alexander Technique focuses on correcting the misalignment and promoting optimal alignment of the head, neck, spine, and torso by examining and correcting the relationships between these critical parts of the body. In a state of optimal alignment, the head releases up and the neck and spine lengthens. The alignment of the head, neck, and spine creates good posture.

The Secrets of Good Posture

Contrary to popular misconception, good posture is not something that you force yourself to do and hold unnaturally. According to the Alexander Technique, engaging in deliberate forced movements and postures is just another way of misusing the body and putting strain on your muscles and internal systems. Rather, good posture develops naturally as you reeducate your body to perform simple tasks—like sitting, standing up, and walking—with greater ease. Performing these tasks correctly involves reeducation in the use of the head, the neck, and the spine. Although the Alexander Technique deals with the whole body, the focus is on the relationships among these three critical parts.

According to Alexander, the spine should be allowed to lengthen and should not be compressed. The lengthening of the spine is key to good posture. Balance is also important. Rather than holding your head stiff and erect to achieve false good posture, it is better to free up the muscles in the neck and allow your head to balance on its own at the top of your spine. The paradox is that good posture is achieved and maintained not by force and discomfort but by ease, balance, and release.

Mental Processes Guide the Physical Changes

Changing how you move and hold your body requires thought. In order to change ingrained body movements and stances, you have to exert mental energy in the forms of paying attention, engaging in detailed self-examination, and visualizing yourself making the corrective actions. Visualizing new, more effective ways to use your body will give you the freedom to choose new, less stressful, and more efficient patterns of movement.

There are other mental forces that drive the bodily changes and make the bodywork effective. These include:

- ଓ Realizing that your movements and posture have become habits.
- ଓ Motivating yourself to break the old patterns and instill new ones.
- ଓ Taking responsibility for behaviors that are under your control if you want to be in control of your life.

THE PROCESS OF REEDUCATION

Reeducation means changing old patterns that do not work for you and establishing new ways of using your body. Learning how to use your body correctly is a process that requires active learning and participation. It is not a process that can be done for you or to you. The guidance provided in Alexander Lessons is designed to reeducate your mind and body in the direction of more efficient movement and posture.

The process of mind-body reeducation in the Alexander Technique can be broken down into the following sequence:

- ଓ Becoming consciously aware of your posture and movements.
- ଓ Learning how to inhibit habitual movement patterns.
- ଓ Consciously using your mind to direct your body to break poor habits.
- ଓ Practicing new movement patterns that are self-enhancing.

EXPERIENCING MODERN ALEXANDER LESSONS

Modern Alexander Lessons, usually taken in a series, are thirty to sixty minutes in length. Although a group format is sometimes used, individual lessons are the norm. In this modality, the giver is called the teacher and the receiver is called the student. As the student, you can learn at your own pace.

The focus is twofold: to discover *how* you move as you perform the tasks related to your everyday life and to help you achieve awareness of the components of those movements. For one person, the movements may involve working at a computer; for another, the movements might be posture and breathing when giving a speech.

The Assessment

Before the educational process can begin, the teacher observes the posture and movement patterns of the student. In addition to the visual examination, the teacher will place his or her hands on the student's neck, back, and shoulder areas in order to assess muscle tension and breathing patterns. The teacher may ask the student to move around or perform simple tasks, like sitting, bending, or walking, as part of the assessment process. The teacher's eyes and hands gather information about the student that will determine the content of the lessons.

The Lesson

Once the assessment is completed, the teacher provides the student, who is comfortably clothed, with verbal instruction and physical guidance, using the hands in a nonintrusive way to coax muscles into better alignment. No movements are forced, and no pain is involved. Concentration and a desire to change are required by the student, whose task it is to relax the body and respond to the teacher's verbal and manual instructions.

Awareness of your movement habits requires using your mind to study what your body has been doing automatically. The next step is to realize that you have the power to change your way of moving. The teacher helps the student achieve awareness by using verbal guidance and gentle, nonmanipulative touch. Once awareness is achieved, you can work toward the goal of learning how to consciously control your movement and make it work for you.

As part of the process, you are guided by the teacher as you engage in the activities that are a part of your life. For example, if you work on a computer many hours of the day, the teacher will guide your movements with gentle touch. If you are a dentist or in another profession that requires leaning over for prolonged periods, the teacher observes and guides you. Your task as the student is to examine your posture and movement patterns while performing the actual activity, inhibit the conditioned patterns of movement that have led to your physical difficulties, and consciously practice more natural ways of using your body.

AN ATTORNEY'S EXPERIENCE WITH ALEXANDER LESSONS

A forty-two-year-old trial lawyer in New York City was frustrated by what she called her "little-girl voice." She felt that her adversaries, particularly the male attorneys, had the edge in court because they could project their voices and capture the attention and respect of the judge and jury. When she tried to project, her voice sounded high-pitched and shrill, rather than rich and resonant. She believed that she was doomed to make a fool of herself and considered changing to a dry branch of law involving no courtroom performances until her massage therapist referred her to a practitioner of the Alexander Technique. After all, Alexander devised his method to correct his own voice projection problem.

During the assessment process, she learned that her body movements were tense and rigid, her posture was forced, and her breathing was shallow, particularly when she was preparing for and participating in a trial. She also tended to pull her shoulders up toward her ears and project her head forward, rather than relaxing her shoulders and allowing her head to float on top of her neck. The posture created by her tense movements and bad habits inhibited the deeper breathing and relaxed muscles required for resonance and projection of one's voice. In other words, she had been tense all the way through school and had been misusing her body for many years. Her "little-girl voice" was the result of habitually poor breathing and tightening of the muscles in her back, neck, and face.

At the end of eight individual Alexander Lessons designed around her goals, the attorney's posture, breathing, confidence, ease of movement, and voice quality and projection all improved. The focus of the lessons was on practicing new movements (as though performing in court), deeper and more steady breathing, and more natural posture. Her ability to see the connection among these various elements has helped her maintain her gains.

BENEFITS OF THE ALEXANDER TECHNIQUE

The Alexander Technique gives you the opportunity to learn how to move with ease and improve your overall functioning. Engaging in this modality releases excess body tension, helps you feel calmer and more confident, enhances your energy and vitality, and increases your powers of concentration on your activities.

By learning to move correctly, you will improve your posture and coordination, heighten your self-awareness, and achieve greater poise and presence. The Alexander Technique is still used today, as it was at the turn of the century, for improved voice projection and resonance. Over the years, famous performers, including actors, musicians, and celebrities, have taken, benefited from, and endorsed Alexander Lessons. Athletes have benefited from Alexander Lessons by learning how to be more graceful and to move with greater ease and efficiency.

The Alexander Technique is a safe method for alleviating stress on the back, the neck, the spine, and the internal organs. It has provided relief from a wide array of physical problems, including chronic back pain; stiff neck and shoulders; work-related upper limb disorder; slipped, herniated, or worn discs; whiplash; sciatica; pinched nerves; scoliosis; hip problems; arthritis; TMJ syndrome; headaches; and angina. This modality has proven to be particularly effective after back surgery to prevent recurrence of the injury.

Because of its value in releasing the musculature, it alleviates respiratory problems, including asthma and emphysema. The Alexander Technique has also been effective in alleviating nervous tension, spastic colon, anxiety, and panic attacks.

Benefits of the Alexander Technique

Easier, more graceful movement.

Better coordination.

Better posture.

Less body tension.

Better voice projection for speaking and singing.

Less pressure on the internal organs and systems.

More energy.

Better concentration.

More self-awareness, self-confidence, and poise.

Reduced risk of recurrence after back surgery.

Freer breathing patterns.

Relief from symptoms of respiratory problems, including asthma and emphysema.

Relief from spastic colon.

Relief from panic attacks.

LESS PAIN AND STRESS FROM:

* Chronic back pain.

* Chronic stiffness and pain in neck and shoulder .

* Work-related upper limb disorder.

* Slipped, herniated, or worn discs.

* Arthritis.

* Scoliosis.

* Hip problems.

* TMJ syndrome.

* Headaches.

* Angina.

* Whiplash.

* Sciatica.

* Pinched nerves.

CHAPTER 20

The Feldenkrais Method

The Feldenkrais Method is an educational approach to body movement that teaches individuals how to move more naturally and efficiently.

According to Feldenkrais, moving your body properly can help you overcome the pain caused by injuries and joint disorders, including TMJ syndrome. Once the new, healthy movement patterns become second nature to you, you will be equipped to prevent the recurrence of old pain patterns and avoid future injuries. In addition to the physical benefits, using your whole body harmoniously can give you more energy and a more favorable view of yourself as a person.

THE HISTORY OF THE FELDENKRAIS METHOD

The Feldenkrais Method was developed by Moshe Feldenkrais, who was born in Russia in 1904. He was a well-traveled and highly educated man. As an adolescent, he traveled to Israel, where he worked as a laborer, a cartographer, and a math tutor. After that, he went to Paris and studied electrical engineering and nuclear science, and earned a doctor-of-science degree from the Sorbonne.

Feldenkrais was active in sports and the martial arts and held a black belt in judo. While playing soccer in England, he suffered a serious, painful knee injury that rendered him unable to walk. His doctors could not promise that surgery would correct the problem.

Creatively using his diverse knowledge of biology, anatomy, physical development, neurology, engineering, and the martial arts, Feldenkrais reeducated his body to move in ways that would alleviate the pain of the knee injury. Using himself as the subject of his evolving method, Feldenkrais taught himself to walk all over again, and he regained complete function in his knee. He believed that an essential part of the process involved tapping into the power of the nervous system.

After his recovery, Feldenkrais studied psychology, neurophysiology, and other disciplines that he thought would shed more light on how he could access and harness the power of the nervous system to improve human functioning. In addition to book learning, he observed the movements of babies and young children in detail. Feldenkrais's wife was a pediatrician, and her practice gave him the opportunity to observe early, natural movements and the factors that sabotage the natural, easy use of the muscles. The Feldenkrais Method recognizes the value of restoring the natural movement patterns that we lost early in life. Feldenkrais was active as a teacher and mentor of his method until his death in 1984.

THE DEVELOPMENT OF MOVEMENT HABITS

According to Feldenkrais, the movement patterns that create and maintain physical pain and mental stress have their roots in childhood. As babies and young children, we develop movement habits that affect our approach to life.

The Feldenkrais Method is designed to correct the poor posture and movement habits that originate early in life. A habit is a behavior that you do compulsively and, in the case of movement, unconsciously. When you engage in any action over and over again, it can become habitual. Being capable of habitual behavior is adaptive, essential to life. If we could not learn to move and perform skills automatically and repeatedly without much thought, we would have to think constantly about doing the simplest things. Imagine having to think about and relearn how to drive a car every time you entered your vehicle. However, as you are well aware, not all habits have positive, healthy consequences. According to Feldenkrais, some of the habitual movement patterns learned early in life are dysfunctional and inefficient and can lead to health problems, physical injury, and low self-esteem.

We develop habitual postural stances and movement patterns by observing and imitating our parents and other role models. Children want to grow up and be like the adults they admire. To accomplish this, children imitate not only the personality traits of those they admire but also the way the role models behave. Physical movement is the most obvious aspect of behavior. For children, the adults' physical qualities, including postural and movement patterns, are more visible, more accessible, and easier to imitate than the adults' inner qualities.

Over time, as you incorporate poor movement habits into all the tasks of daily living, you become used to your twisted, overcompensating, inefficient patterns of movement. You do not realize that moving inappropriately is causing you pain. This lack of awareness results in your accepting discomfort as a normal part of daily life. If you take your pain for granted and learn to live with it, what else might you begin to take for granted and learn to tolerate?

The Feldenkrais Method can help you become aware of long-standing unconscious patterns of movement that are limiting, inefficient, and contradictory. Just because you have been doing something a particular way for many years does not mean that you cannot change it. If what you are doing is causing pain, it is worth making the commitment to change it.

WHY CHANGE HOW YOU MOVE?

Why take the time to analyze and change how you move and how you perform simple tasks? According to Feldenkrais, discarding strained, inefficient movement patterns and learning to use your whole body in a synergistic, integrated way can lead to personal growth, an enhanced self-image, and a better life.

Feldenkrais conceived of self-image as consisting of four parts: movement, sensation, feeling, and thought. All four aspects interact with each other in every action we take. They are intertwined, and they affect each other. For example, feeling angry triggers negative and tense bodily sensations and thoughts. The angry feelings and associated bodily sensations and negative thoughts rigidify your posture and tense the muscles of your face, your jaw, and the rest of your body, resulting in tense and unnatural movement. Another example is that negative thoughts about yourself as a person will trigger depressed and anxious feelings, uncomfortable sensations (like physical tension), strained movements, and perhaps hunched posture. Improving your self-image can begin with any of its four elements. Entering anywhere into the system with a healthy approach will have a positive ripple effect on the remaining components and improve functioning as a whole.

Feldenkrais believed that changing self-image would be best accomplished by changing the *movement* component of action. Why? For one thing, the nervous system is more occupied with movement than with sensations, feelings, or thoughts. Feldenkrais reasoned that changing the feature that has the most nervous-system involvement would lead to the deepest level of overall change.

Another reason Feldenkrais focused on movement is that it is the only component of the system that is directly observable and measurable. You cannot see sensations, feelings, and thoughts, and, therefore, they are more difficult to examine, discuss, and change. It is only by bringing something into awareness and by studying it that you can begin to improve it.

Yet another reason that movement is a critical aspect of your functioning is that how you feel when you move your muscles is a barometer of how the rest of you is doing. Many people remain unaware of their sensations, thoughts, and feelings until their impact reaches the muscles. Your attitude and whole being are affected by the state of the muscles. Tense, overused muscles make you work harder physically and mentally. The continual drain on your energy makes you tired and irritable, conditions that can snowball into depression. Working on movement directly can be the key to shifting this negative pattern into achieving personal growth. Greater ease and efficiency of movement allows the muscles to work properly, with less strain, and allows for more efficient expenditure of your energy. Under these conditions, the other three components of self-image—sensations, feelings, and thoughts—will also be experienced more positively. When you have balanced and pleasant bodily sensations, balanced and positive feelings, and rational, confident thoughts, you experience good self-esteem and mental health.

SOMATIC EDUCATION FOR CHANGING HOW YOU MOVE

Unlearning old patterns and replacing them with new patterns takes motivation, active participation, and practice, the components of any successful educational experience. In the context of bodywork, learning new ways of using your body is known as *somatic education*.

Somatic education involves learning how to take charge of those aspects of your bodily functioning that are under your control. The Feldenkrais Method is a form of somatic education that uses gentle movement to retrain the central nervous system so that you can change poor movement patterns and increase your repertoire of movements. The Feldenkrais Method offers new choices to replace the old patterns.

The Feldenkrais Method is not something that is done to you. Rather, it is a learning experience. It is a system, rather than a treatment.

According to Edward Feldman, a chiropractor trained in the Feldenkrais Method, Feldenkrais is based on a systemic model rather than a medical model. Unlike the medical model, which is static and based on diagnosis, this systemic model is fluid and educationally oriented.

What makes the Feldenkrais Method of somatic education unique is the emphasis on bringing into conscious awareness detailed aspects of your unconscious patterns of movement. It is only through recognizing in depth how you move your body that you can begin to make changes. According to Feldenkrais, when you become aware of how you move, your movements become under your control. Your awareness of and emerging sense of control over your movements will help you learn how to restore healthy patterns of movement.

As you progress, messages will be sent by your muscles through your nervous system to inform your brain that your body is using its muscles more efficiently, with less strain and less tension. Through this neural feedback, new connections will be established between the body and the brain that will improve your overall physical and mental functioning. The discarding of harmful movement habits and the learning and practicing of the new movement patterns establish efficiency and harmony throughout the systems of the body and brain. Your more fluid movements and more relaxed muscles will help release long-standing pain patterns. Overall health and homeostasis are facilitated by the more appropriate movement patterns. Incorporating the learning into your daily life can help avoid future pain and physical injury.

Somatic education in this modality begins with becoming aware of your movements and their smaller components. For example, think about and observe what you do when changing from a seated to a standing position. According to Feldenkrais, most people overestimate the amount of physical effort needed to accomplish the task. We tend to stiffen the muscles in the back of the neck in anticipation of the movement. Then, we use the bottoms of our feet to push down on the floor before the rest of the body is ready to follow. This motion is inefficient and does not allow for the distribution of effort so much a part of smooth, flowing movement. Efficient movement flows fluidly through the skeleton, from joint to joint, using the proper amount of exertion at each point.

FORMATS OF MOVEMENT LESSONS

There are two formats available for the movement lessons of the Feldenkrais Method: (1) Functional Integration lessons, which are private, one-on-one sessions tailored to your needs, and (2) Awareness Through Movement classes taught in a group setting. In both formats, you are fully dressed in loose, comfortable clothing. No oil is used.

The exercises and movements learned in both formats can be practiced and mentally rehearsed as you perform your daily activities. It is the incorporation of the new movement patterns into your everyday life that will help you break old movement habits.

Functional Integration Lessons

Functional Integration lessons are thirty- to sixty-minute individual bodywork sessions. In the Feldenkrais Method, the practitioner is considered a teacher and the client a student. It is the task of the teacher to create optimal conditions for learning and change to occur, thereby expanding the student's perception of choice. The teacher will make the learning experience comfortable for you and will tailor the lessons to suit your individual needs.

As the student, you are instructed to sit or lie on a padded bodywork table. The area of injury, pain, or discomfort is not necessarily manipulated directly. Rather, the teacher observes your movement patterns and then addresses those patterns that are causing the problem. The teacher might ask you to move your head and other parts of your body in certain directions in order to assess your range of motion, flexibility, blockages of movement, and movement habits.

Your movements are analyzed and studied by you and your Feldenkrais teacher in detail. Then, correct movements are practiced and mentally rehearsed over time. Inefficient, energy-draining, and strained movement patterns will be brought to your attention both verbally and through the teacher's gentle touch. Suggested new movements are never forced. The teacher's touch is a form of tactile, kinesthetic communication that is used as a vehicle to communicate new choices you can make when moving your body.

Functional Integration lessons teach you to relieve chronic pain and reduce the strain on your muscles by changing the way you move your body while engaging in your regular activities. You will learn to become aware of the stress you are putting on your muscles. You will be taught how not to stress your muscles and how to stop causing yourself pain by learning more efficient, harmonious movement patterns that you can integrate into your daily activities. As the new movement patterns take hold, you will experience greater energy and freedom.

Awareness Through Movement Lessons

Awareness Through Movement lessons are done in a group format. Each group lesson lasts between thirty and sixty minutes. The teacher uses slow and gentle movement, which allows the students to find their own way during the lesson. The lessons move gradually from very simple to more complex movements.

Techniques are used to help the students become aware of their bodily movements as an important step toward change. All students are respected at their individual level of mastery, and no one is pushed beyond points of resistance.

There are literally hundreds of Awareness Through Movement lessons and exercises. A recent outgrowth of the original Feldenkrais Awareness Through Movement lessons is Relaxercise, a movement exercise system based on the interconnection of the brain and the muscles. Relaxercise consists of simple exercises designed to enable the brain and nervous system to release muscular tension, increase flexibility, improve poor posture, and change dysfunctional movement patterns. Relaxercise focuses on correcting unhealthy sitting postures, a major cause of chronic muscle pain.

BENEFITS OF THE FELDENKRAIS METHOD

This form of somatic education is beneficial on many levels of functioning. Becoming aware of your movement patterns is the first step toward alleviating a host of physical and self-image problems.

On the physical level, the benefits of the Feldenkrais Method affect both observable and internal processes. Your body will move more freely, your posture will improve, and your physical performance will be more fluid. You will be able to do the tasks of daily living more efficiently, with a wider range of motion, and with less muscle strain. Your muscles will become less tense, and you can will experience relief from back, neck, and shoulder pain. The Feldenkrais Method also relieves headaches, jaw pain, and joint pain, including the pain of TMJ syndrome and carpal tunnel syndrome. Once you incorporate the new movement patterns into your daily life, you will be in a better position to prevent the recurrence of these painful conditions and to avoid future injuries.

As you relax the muscles in your chest and diaphragm, you will be able to breathe more deeply and easily. More oxygen will enter your lungs and your brain. Improved breathing patterns and increased oxygenation of cells promote vitality and energy.

Breaking unhealthy movement habits and replacing them with correct patterns can lead to greater ease of movement, grace, flexibility, and coordination. Athletes, musicians, and actors have refined their performances through the Feldenkrais Method.

Your improved movement patterns trigger pleasant body sensations, creative thinking, and positive emotions. Your ability to manage your stress will be enhanced. Some individuals report experiencing the rebirth of the openness, creativity, and spontaneity they possessed as a child.

Being more in control of your bodily movement and feeling more comfortable as you move through the world provide a foundation for feeling more in control of your life. When you feel optimistic and in charge of your life, you will be motivated to reach your potential as a human being.

THE FELDENKRAIS GUILD

Training programs in the Feldenkrais Method must be approved by the Feldenkrais Guild in order for practitioners of this modality to use the service marks of Feldenkrais, Functional Integration, and Awareness Through Movement. The guild was established by Moshe Feldenkrais in 1977 and is the official organization of Feldenkrais Method practitioners. Courses are offered internationally in an intensive program encompassing more than 160 days of training in a four-year period. Training is based on the theories and teachings of Moshe Feldenkrais. There are currently more than seven hundred certified Feldenkrais practitioners in the United States. No specific background is required for admission to the guild's training program. Training in the Feldenkrais Method at the guild has attracted chiropractors who want to look more deeply at the movement patterns underlying their clients' pain syndromes.

Benefits of the Feldenkrais Method

Greater freedom and flexibility of movement.

Improved posture.

More fluid physical performance.

More efficient performance of the tasks of daily living.

Wider range of motion.

Less muscle strain and less tension.

Relief from back, neck, and shoulder pain.

Relief from headaches, jaw pain, and joint pain.

Relief from the pain of such conditions as TMJ syndrome
    and carpal tunnel syndrome.

Less frequent recurrence of these painful conditions.

Reduced risk of future physical injuries.

Improved breathing patterns.

Renewed vitality and energy.

More graceful movement and better coordination.

Refined performance for athletes, musicians, and actors.

Triggering of pleasant body sensations, creative thinking,
    and positive emotions.

Enhanced ability to manage stress.

Rebirth of the openness, creativity, and spontaneity
    possessed as a child.

Increased feeling of control over one's life.

Greater motivation to reach one's potential as a human being.

Healing with Energy

Reiki

Polarity Therapy

Therapeutic Touch

Although Reiki and other energy methods, including Polarity Therapy and Therapeutic Touch, appear to operate on principles very different from those on which other types of massage therapy and bodywork are based, they play a significant and growing role in physical and mental health.

Reiki is the best known, and perhaps most mysterious, of the bodywork modalities that use life energy for healing.

Polarity Therapy supplements healing energy with nutritional suggestions and exercise.

Western science had shown little interest in researching the healing power of life energy until the development of Therapeutic Touch—a bodywork modality in which, paradoxically, healing is achieved with no physical touch.

CHAPTER 21

Reiki

Reiki is a Japanese word that translates as "universal life energy," the power which resides in all living matter. The syllable *rei* refers to the universal, boundless aspect of this energy, whereas *ki* is the life force, which flows through all living beings. *Ki* is named *chi* by the Chinese and *prana* by the Hindus.

Reiki, when activated and applied for the purpose of healing, addresses the body, mind, and spirit, as well as the relationships among them. Reiki accelerates the body's ability to heal physical ailments and opens the mind and spirit to the causes of disease and pain. The emphasis in Reiki is on taking responsibility for your life and the joys of balanced wellness.

Reiki is a gentle hands-on approach that addresses your energy field as a means of healing wounds and pain on all levels—physical, mental, emotional, and spiritual—so that you can feel healthy and free of blockages. The roots of Reiki go back to the ancient origins of natural healing. In fact, the origins of Reiki have been traced back more than twenty-five hundred years to the ancient Tibetan sutras.

THE REDISCOVERY OF REIKI

In other bodywork modalities, theories and techniques begin with ideas and talents that individuals have developed into cohesive systems over time. Reiki is different. Reiki was rediscovered.

Mikao Usui, Ph.D., is the recognized founder of Reiki as a healing method. He rediscovered the use of universally available forces to bring people into gentle contact with their sources of pain and disease. There is no known written record of Usui's rediscovery of an ancient approach to healing. However, Hawayo Takata, the third Reiki master, related the history orally to her students, who kept it alive throughout the generations.

Usui was born in Japan in the middle of the nineteenth century. He was fascinated with Buddhism and wanted to learn how to apply the Buddha's ability to heal people suffering from illness. He became a doctor of philosophy and, in the late 1800s, a professor at Doshisha University, a Christian school in Kyoto, Japan. Challenged by his students to demonstrate the healing powers used by the great spiritual leaders of the world, Usui left the school to embark on an intensive search for the secrets of healing.

He spent time in the United States studying in Chicago, and he traveled throughout Japan, where he studied at Buddhist temples to find answers to his questions about healing. He spoke with Buddhist teachers, priests, and monks, who all told him that there once was a system of Buddhist healing that was now lost, and that the Buddhist ability to heal was lost with the information. Along his journey, Usui learned Chinese and Sanskrit so that he could read the ancient documents. He eventually discovered the formula for healing in the Tibetan sutras, ancient Buddhist texts written in Sanskrit.

Knowing the formula was not enough. For Usui, obtaining healing power was a complex spiritual experience that included fasting and meditating for twenty-one days on top of a holy mountain. The healing power was presented to him as a vision of light entering his consciousness. Usui was initiated in this way as the first Reiki master, the Grand Master.

Usui returned home to Japan, where he practiced Reiki for the rest of his life. He had the perspective that unless he passed on the healing power, Reiki would be lost again.

THE SUCCESSION OF REIKI MASTERS

A Reiki master is an individual who has healing power through the unblocked access to universal life energy. The Reiki master channels the universal life energy to the receiver of Reiki. You can only become a Reiki master through a series of attunements provided by a Reiki master. The series of attunements imparts the healing power of the master to the student in such a way that the student becomes a Reiki master who can then heal and teach others.

Usui chose Chujiro Hayashi in 1925 to succeed him as the Grand Master so that the healing power of Reiki could be preserved and taught to others. Through a series of attunements and by absorbing the teachings of Reiki, Hayashi became the second Reiki master. He opened the first Reiki clinic in Tokyo for the treatment of severely ill individuals. In order to continue the preservation of Reiki, Hayashi initiated thirteen Reiki masters.

The thirteenth was Hawayo Takata, who is known for introducing Reiki to the West.

It was Hawayo Takata's desire to be cured of a serious illness that took her on a journey from her home in Hawaii to Hayashi's Reiki clinic in Japan. She was treated by two Reiki practitioners each day. She reported that she could feel the heat of the energy coming from their hands so strongly that she thought it was generated by a machine. She became familiar with Reiki as a receiver, and when she was cured of her illnesses, her strong desire to become a Reiki master was fulfilled.

In 1937, Takata returned to Hawaii, and Hayashi and his family helped her establish Reiki there. Between 1970 and 1980, Takata initiated twenty-two Reiki masters. These twenty-two teachers have taught others through-out the world. It is estimated that there are currently about five thousand Reiki masters and half a million people practicing Reiki.

HOW REIKI PROMOTES HEALING

Exactly how Reiki works from a scientific perspective is not really known. However, many receivers of Reiki have obtained significant relief.

The theory underlying how Reiki works places an emphasis on the intricate and reciprocal relationships among body, mind, and spirit. According to the Reiki masters, we are alive because life force is flowing through our bodies by means of pathways called chakras, meridians, and nadis. The life energy also flows around each of us in a field of energy called the aura. The life force nourishes the organs and cells of the body, supporting them in their vital functions, by flowing through these pathways. When this flow is disrupted, the organs and tissues of the body become less efficient and badly affected.

According to the theory of Reiki, all of us are born with the potential to access this universal life energy, which maintains our health and a balanced internal state. The flow of the life force is influenced by our thoughts and feelings. As we go through life, we are influenced by experiences that disrupt and taint our thoughts and feelings about ourselves and the world. As we begin to accept these negative thoughts and feelings on both conscious and unconscious levels, our systems become weakened, and our access to the universal life energy becomes blocked.

Reiki masters are empowered to unblock the energy pathways in others, allowing the universal life force to flow through them. The healing power of Reiki resides in the flow of Reiki energy through the channel (the giver) to the opened pathways of the receiver.

Once the energy is received, it must be empowered by the receiver in order to work effectively. In this sense, the receiver plays an active role in creating health, inner harmony, and balance. The conscious decision to participate in one's self-improvement is the active commitment to Reiki that makes it a complete system. This commitment to one's own healing is at the heart of the Reiki ideals. These ideals comprise the ethical principles of Reiki and serve as guidelines for a gracious, fulfilling life.

EXPERIENCING REIKI

Reiki is a gentle but powerful bodywork modality. A Reiki session lasts anywhere from sixty to ninety minutes. The receiver is fully clothed, and no oil is used. The Reiki energy enters the giver through the top of the head and exits through the hands, where it is directed into the body or energy field of the receiver (see Figure 21.1).

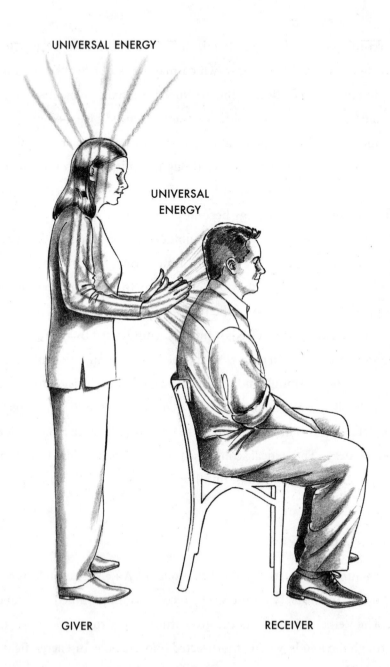

UNIVERSAL ENERGY

UNIVERSAL
ENERGY

GIVER

RECEIVER

Figure 21.1   The Flow of Universal Energy from Giver to Receiver

The Reiki Ideals

Just for today.

I will let go of anger.

I will let go of worry.

I will give thanks for my many blessings.

I will do my work honestly.

I will be kind to my neighbor and every living being.

The practitioner directs and concentrates the energy by placing his or her hands on ten to twenty specific areas of the receiver's body to cause the negative energy to break apart and dissipate. The hand positions are chosen to impact the chakras and the internal organs and glands of the receiver. Each hand position is maintained for several minutes to allow the receiver time to draw on it.

In addition to having a planned approach, the practitioner also relies on intuition and feedback from the receiver's aura when selecting particular areas of the body for treatment. As the receiver draws on the channeled energy, healing is facilitated by the increasing flow of ki through the affected parts of the energy field, charging them with positive energy. The giver raises the vibratory level of the energy field in and around the body where the negative thoughts and feelings have become attached. Through this energy transmission from giver to receiver, Reiki clears and heals the receiver's energy pathways, allowing the life force to flow in a healthy and natural way, uninterrupted by blockages that have now been removed.

An unusual aspect of this modality is that the receiver does not even have to be present to experience the healing powers of Reiki. According to the theory underlying Reiki, natural laws exist that allow for the transfer of life energy over distance to one or more receivers at a time. For a long-distance session, an appointment of about fifteen to twenty minutes is made, and a photograph of the receiver is used to help channel the energy. The receiver is advised to sit or lie down during the appointed time in order to be ready to receive the treatment and feel the flow of energy.

Not everyone has the same reaction to a Reiki session. Some feel more in tune with their inner selves. Some feel unconditional love from the universe. Some have interesting sensory experiences. Some feel a renewal of their spirit. The most widely experienced reaction to Reiki is a feeling of profound relaxation.

A MASSAGE THERAPIST GIVES AND RECEIVES REIKI

Adrienne Rodewald has both given and received Reiki. She views Reiki as "wonderful to use on people after they recover from surgery or when they are in a diseased or compromised physical condition. Or if someone is in grief. Massage can be too intense."

Adrienne believes that "Reiki allows a lot of healing to go on. It allows the exchange of positive and negative energy in the body. Reiki promotes healing." Adrienne has used Reiki on clients with fractures and with cancer. In the case of fractures and other injuries, Adrienne believes that healing was faster than if Reiki had not been used. In the case of cancer, even though Reiki is not a cure, clients feel better after receiving it.

Adrienne has received Reiki before having hospital procedures done.

"I've done the complete Reiki session. It takes an hour to receive, that is, the front and the back of the body. There's absolutely no talking. It's very relaxing." She believes that she has been more relaxed facing these procedures and has healed more quickly when receiving Reiki.

THE BENEFITS OF REIKI

Reiki supports the body's natural ability to heal itself, minimizes your sense of helplessness when facing disease or trauma, and brings your body back into harmony by relieving physical, spiritual, and emotional blockages. Reiki helps alleviate the discomfort caused by aches and pains, stress, anxiety, grief, depression, and life changes. Increased energy and vitality, a strengthened immune system, accelerated healing, the cleansing of bodily toxins, and improved overall health are associated with Reiki. For some, Reiki awakens creativity, enhances intuition, and provides the internal motivation to make better choices regarding mental, physical, and spiritual health.

Reiki can be applied to people of all ages because it is a universal system, encompassing all living beings. When Reiki is applied by a parent, a benefit for infants and young children is the intensification of the bonding between parent and child. Infants and children can thrive when given universal life energy. The process can help keep their pathways open throughout the course of development, allowing for continual renewal of the body, mind, and spirit.

This gentle modality is pleasant to receive and does not involve manipulation of muscle tissues. It is safe for most individuals. However, to be on the safe side, sessions should be shortened when Reiki is applied to very young children, to the geriatric population, or to seriously ill individuals.

The Benefits of Reiki

Support of the body's natural ability to heal itself.

Reduced sense of helplessness when facing disease or trauma.

Return of harmony within the body.

Relief from physical, spiritual, and emotional blockages.

Less discomfort caused by aches and pains, stress, anxiety, grief, depression, and life changes.

More energy and vitality.

Less stress.

Stronger immune system.

Accelerated healing.

Elimination of toxins.

Better overall health.

More creativity.

Better intuition.

Stronger internal motivation to make better choices regarding mental, physical, and spiritual health.

It can be applied to people of all ages.

It can be done long-distance.

When applied by a parent, it promotes bonding between parent and child.

It is safe for most individuals.

It promotes the health of animals and plants.

Even though Reiki has a spiritual foundation, it is not a religion. No particular belief system is required on the part of the receiver for Reiki to be effective. The infants and young children who benefit from Reiki have not yet formed a belief system or a commitment to a religion. The lack of necessity of believing in Reiki is further evidenced by the use of Reiki with animals and plants. According to Reiki, universal life energy flows not only through human beings but through all living things.

Reiki is not considered a cure-all. Rather, Reiki is the modern application of an ancient healing art that acts by harnessing and channeling the life energy around us for the purpose of facilitating health and well-being. This modality can be used as a safe adjunct to psychotherapeutic and medical treatments.

CHAPTER 22

Polarity Therapy

Polarity Therapy is a form of energy work that synthesizes ancient Eastern and contemporary Western concepts. This approach was developed in the mid-1920s by Randolph Stone, a chiropractor, an osteopath, and an herbalist.

Polarity Therapy offers a self-contained system for healing and maintaining good health. The system consists of bodywork, nutritional suggestions, and exercises. Bodywork is at the heart of the Polarity system. It takes the form of subtle touches and gentle holding on specific points of the body. The goal of the touching is to harmonize the flow of energy through the body and to enhance the body's internal balance.

ANCIENT KNOWLEDGE IN A MODERN CONTEXT

Randolph Stone was born in Austria in 1890. As a young man, he emigrated to Chicago, where he studied chiropractic, osteopathic, and naturopathic medicine. Stone's goal was to find the underlying reasons why proper diet and exercise promote good health. He also wanted to understand why individuals differ in their degree of health and vitality.

His questions motivated him to study Chinese acupuncture, herbal medicine, and the medicine of ancient Middle Eastern and Indian cultures. This contemporary bodywork modality has its origins in Ayurveda, an ancient mind-body healing art that originated in India more than five thousand years ago.

Stone focused on two beliefs that he uncovered in the ancient writings. The first is that life energy permeates the body and keeps it healthy. The second is that obstructions to the flow of life energy contribute to disease. These became the guiding principles of Polarity Therapy.

Stone spent many years in India studying meditation and practicing the freeing of life energy. He was trying to apply his synthesis of ancient and contemporary theory to the practice of healing.

Stone's theory of healing is a modern conceptualization of the ancient Eastern concept of chakras and life energy. In developing Polarity Therapy, he combined these ancient teachings with contemporary electromagnetic theory. It is the juxtaposition of ancient healing with modern science that makes Polarity Therapy unique.

THE FLOW OF ENERGY

Stone developed Polarity Therapy on the premise that the universe consists of a vital force, known as energy, that flows around and through everyone. This energy must flow freely, without encountering blockages, and at a consistent pace if the body is to be balanced and to function efficiently.

Stone theorized that natural healing techniques like proper nutrition and exercise are effective because they stimulate and maintain the balanced, unblocked flow of life energy through the body. It is the balanced and free flow of life energy around and within you that creates harmony in and among your physical body, your thoughts, your emotions, and your behavior. When your energy is balanced and flowing freely, you have a better chance of maintaining good health and reducing your physical and mental tension.

According to Stone, the flow of life energy through this system is influenced by the poles of the cells throughout the body. Polarity Therapy is based on the principle that every cell in the body has both negative and positive poles. Life energy is in constant pulsation from positive to negative poles via a neutral position, creating fields and energetic lines of force.

Stone conceptualized healing as balancing the energy flow throughout a system of lines of force running horizontally, vertically, and diagonally throughout the body. Stone believed that this energy system of fields and lines creates an energetic template for the body. He called this template "the wireless anatomy of man."

Stone placed within the wireless anatomy five centers, or chakras, each with its own location and each governing a different aspect of our internal functioning.

In ancient Eastern history, chakras were conceived as centers in the body that have life energy flowing through them.

In Figure 22.1, the five centers, or chakras, are named for the five elements of life energy in the universe that Stone read about in India: earth, water, fire, air, and ether.

- *Earth chakra* governs the elimination of waste products.
- *Water chakra* governs glandular activity and motivation.
- *Fire chakra* governs digestion.
- *Air chakra* governs circulation, heart, and lungs.
- *Ether chakra* governs voice, hearing, and throat. The ether element is the most subtle of the energies and has the highest frequency of vibration. It is the place with no positive or negative pole.

According to the theory of Polarity Therapy, freeing the flow of energy through the chakras creates harmony within the wireless anatomy of man. Polarity Therapy is designed to balance the energy currents through the complex, interconnected system.

By placing the hands on the targeted areas of the body, the Polarity therapist redirects the flow of energy to where it is needed. As the energy becomes redirected, it creates new currents in the body. The new currents are free to flow in any direction in the body without following the lines of the wireless map of man created by Stone.

When the energy flows freely, the system becomes balanced and achieves homeostasis, or a steady state. A homeostatic, unblocked system helps the body become stronger and better able to defend against illness. Achieving homeostasis also reduces stress and promotes feelings of well-being.

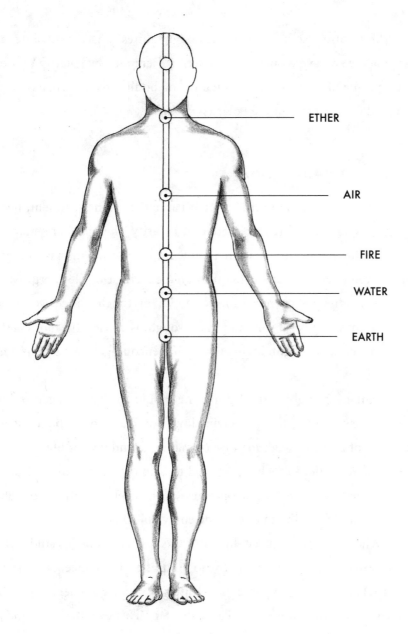

ETHER

AIR

FIRE

WATER

EARTH

Figure 22.1   Locations of Chakras in the Body

Stone also recognized that the body requires consistent maintenance. Keeping the energy flowing and balanced is facilitated by Polarity Yoga exercises, proper diet, and the elimination of bodily toxins. That is why he included these factors in the Polarity work.

POLARITY THERAPY TODAY

When Randolph Stone retired, Pierre Pannetier, Stone's student, became the spokesperson and representative of Polarity Therapy. Pannetier was a naturopathic physician. He is credited with putting an emphasis on gentle touch. Pannetier recognized that the depth of release of life energy was not necessarily directly correlated with depth of touch. Since we are surrounded by energy and it is running through us constantly, blockages can be addressed with a light, loving touch that encourages, rather than forces, energy flow.

Pannetier taught that this touching should be given in a gentle, loving way. He viewed giving touch as giving love, not in any romantic sense but in the sense of love thy neighbor, love of mankind, and love of life. The loving nature of Pannetier's touch is intended to help the client trust and become open to the healing work. The openness of the client's attitude contributes to the therapist's ability to release the energy blockages.

When Pannetier retired, his work was carried on by his student, Alan Siegel, a naturopathic physician who simplified the concepts underlying Polarity Therapy. He compared the release and balance of energy in the body to recharging a car battery. Like Pannetier, Siegel believes that light and gentle touch is sufficient to get your life energy flowing.

EXPERIENCING THE POLARITY THERAPY SYSTEM

Polarity Therapy is a holistic modality, usually given in a series of four sessions. A Polarity Therapy program includes bodywork focused on restoring your energetic balance, a recommended set of Polarity exercises, and guidelines for proper diet tailored to your needs.

Bodywork

For bodywork, the client wears underwear or loose, comfortable clothing. The client is draped with a sheet. No oil or lotion is used. Bodywork sessions are generally sixty to ninety minutes in length.

During bodywork sessions, the body is gently manipulated in order to enhance the energy flow. The practitioner uses light and deep touches, rhythmic pressing, gentle rocking, and stretching to balance the body's subtle energy fields. The therapist always uses both hands, either resting gently on a part of your body or engaging in movements. Each hand touches a pole, one positive and one negative, and rests on these areas lightly as a means of balancing and releasing your energy.

Not all Polarity therapists use exactly the same touches or the same depth of touch. Typical modes of touch include rocking and rhythmically pressing different areas at various depths. There are many poles mapped out in the wireless anatomy and many ways for the therapist to approach each area. The theory behind the therapy inspired a wide array of choices. In any particular session, some areas might need more attention than others. The touches are tailored to your needs as determined by prior discussion with the Polarity therapist and the feedback your body gives the therapist, who is constantly examining your individual energy patterns.

Polarity Exercises

The exercises, to be done between sessions and to incorporate into your life if you wish, are based on Yoga positions. Maintaining the Yoga postures helps you unblock and balance your vital energy. The Polarity therapist will select exercises suitable to your needs and show you how to do them.

Different Yoga positions are aimed at freeing energy at the various chakras or energy centers throughout the body. Polarity Therapy includes Yoga-based exercises that help improve the internal functioning of your body as well as your mental state. The exercises vary in focus from establishing healthy breathing patterns and clearing the sinuses to improving elimination to balancing your right and left brain.

To get a flavor of the nature of Polarity exercise, look at the squat postures depicted in Figures 22.2, 22.3, and 22.4. The squat posture is only one of the many Polarity exercises available. We are highlighting it here because it is a simple exercise for you to try, and trying it will give you an idea whether you would like to know more. Look at the illustrations as you read how to do this Polarity exercise.

After assuming the position depicted in Figure 22.2, rock your body gently, back and forth for about a minute, and then side to side for about the same amount of time. Then slowly wrap your arms around your knees as you gently push your knees together with your arms, as shown in Figure 22.3. While in this second squat position, take a deep breath and let it out while making a sound. Bend your head slightly forward to increase relaxation surrounding the earth chakra. Rock back and forth and from side to side, as you did in the first squat position.

In the third squat position, shown in Figure 22.4, you can move your feet apart a little more, as long as no movement is forced. Make sure your

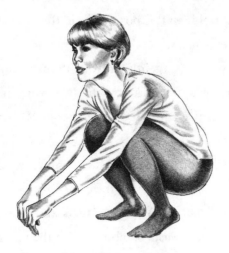

Figure 22.2   The Squat Position (First)

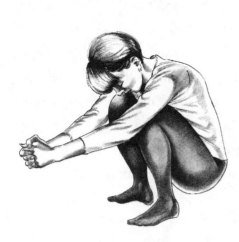

Figure 22.3   The Squat Position (Second)

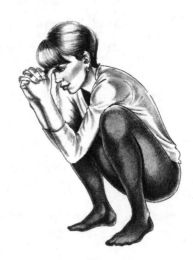

Figure 22.4   The Squat Position (Third)

body becomes comfortable in this position, and then move your knees out-ward with your upper arms, which, as you can see, are placed between your knees. You can rest your head gently on your thumbs, which are placed as shown. Now you are ready to rock your body as you did in the first two squat positions. The entire squat sequence should take you less than five minutes to complete.

The squat postures target the movement and renewal of energy in the earth chakra. At the same time, the squatting postures can facilitate the elim-ination of gas and other bodily waste products and increase the intake of oxygen. The elimination of waste combined with the renewal and alertness associated with an oxygenated brain can produce feelings of harmony and well-being. The squat exercises also strengthen the back and spine, alleviate stress, and can help you sleep.

Nutritional Suggestions

Stone was ahead of his time in realizing the impact of the good and bad chemicals that we consume. He believed that food has energetic properties that influence the functioning of the body centers and the flow of life energy. Just as certain foods can block and otherwise inhibit the flow of energy, other foods can correct imbalances and help maintain balance. He catego-rized food by its relationship to the five elements (earth, water, fire, air, ether) and made recommendations based on each individual's needs. Stone typically recommended a vegetarian diet and daily flushing of the system through the use of natural herbs.

A CONVERTED SKEPTIC

Adrienne Rodewald, a massage therapist, was skeptical about Polarity when she studied it from books. It was only when she experienced it that she was convinced of its impact. "It was just a 'Wow! What happened?' What happened was I felt I was literally floating, literally coming off the table. I could have read about that for ten years and never have believed it. Once I experienced it, that was it. I was sold on the benefits of it."

Adrienne incorporates Polarity into an eclectic massage that also includes Swedish massage and trigger-point therapy. She leaves three to five minutes at the end of the massage for Polarity. During that time, she places her left hand behind the client's shoulder blades and her right hand over the sacrum. There is no talking. Adrienne says that she can feel the transfer of energy through the change in the temperature of her hands. She recalled one session in which her right hand got so warm that she had to remove it from the area she was touching.

The client Adrienne felt received the most benefit from Polarity was a male in his thirties who arrived for his first massage very tense and wired. He grabbed the edges of the massage table as though he was holding on for dear life. Adrienne told him that he could relax, but he didn't know how. "So we had to really work through that for several sessions—just getting him to relax. One day, I thought I would try Polarity on him. He had the same experience I had of feeling as though he were floating. After that, he never wanted to end the massage without Polarity. For him and many others, Polarity has to be part of the massage no matter what else happens."

THE BENEFITS OF POLARITY THERAPY

As the flow of energy becomes more properly balanced, emotional tension and physical pain are released. When your energy is balanced, you feel more energetic and less tired. The muscular tension throughout your body will be reduced.

When energy pathways are opened, stress is released and circulation, respiration, and elimination are improved. The immune system functions more efficiently. The strengthening of the immune system helps prevent illness and helps you heal more quickly from illness and injury.

Because Polarity works with the energy moving through the body, mind, and emotions, its benefits go beyond the physical. Mental health benefits include decreased mental tension, increased self-awareness, and emotional vitality. The emotional vitality derives from the releasing of emotional patterns that have maintained a negative hold on you. Negative emotional patterns reside not only in the mind but in the body as well.

Doing the recommended exercises and using the nutritional suggestions made by the Polarity therapist will enhance your bodily awareness and self-esteem. The exercises can improve your breathing patterns, reduce muscle tension, help remove toxins from the body, and help you sleep. Remember that Polarity is a system that begins with bodywork. Taking good care of your body as you go through the course of each day is what will help you reap the most benefits from Polarity Therapy or from any form of bodywork.

Benefits of Polarity Therapy

The balancing of life energy.

The release of emotional and muscular tension.

Lessening of physical pain.

Reduced pain in back and neck.

Relief from migraine headaches.

Relief from menstrual pain and discomfort.

Increased energy.

Less fatigue.

Less stress.

Improved respiration.

Clear sinuses.

Better circulation.

Better digestion and elimination.

Better elimination of waste products and toxins.

More efficient functioning of immune system.

Less risk of illness.

Faster healing from illness and injury.

Decreased mental tension.

Improved quality of sleep.

Relief from negative emotional patterns.

Enhanced self-awareness and self-esteem.

CHAPTER 23

Therapeutic Touch

Therapeutic Touch is a safe and gentle body-work approach. The name is a little misleading because, in this modality, direct touching of the skin is not necessary for positive results. It is an energy-based therapy, rather than a form of massage therapy. What is manipulated by the practitioner is the invisible energy field surrounding the body, not the body tissue itself.

Therapeutic Touch practitioners are called healers, and the clients are called healees. The goal of the healer is to facilitate the integration of the body, mind, and spirit of the healee.

THE SIGNIFICANCE OF THE ENERGY FIELD

The theory and practice of Therapeutic Touch is based on the principle that a human energy field, which is electromagnetic in nature, extends beyond the skin and surrounds the entire body. Energy is conceived as flowing from the environment around us, through the human energy system, exiting back into the environment, then through the human energy system again, constantly replenishing us in a cyclical fashion. The energy, as it flows through us, travels through a complex system of bodily networks, analogous to the meridians depicted in traditional Chinese medicine.

Within the context of the Therapeutic Touch modality, when you are healthy and intact, your energy field is abundant, well-organized, and flows in balanced patterns. Illness, disease, injuries, wounds, and negative feeling-states are viewed as creating imbalances, disorganization, and depletion of the human energy field. The practice of Therapeutic Touch is designed to fight acute illness and heal wounds by balancing, organizing, and replenishing your energy field when you are suffering from illness or injury.

This relatively new practice is derived from several ancient healing practices, including the laying on of hands. The concepts of life energy and healing through restoring and balancing life energy have been a part of Eastern cultures for thousands of years. It is only recently that Western cultures have begun to embrace the idea that life energy exists and plays an important role in our state of health and feelings of well-being.

THE DEVELOPMENT OF
THE THERAPEUTIC TOUCH MODALITY

The contemporary practice of Therapeutic Touch was developed in the 1970s by Dolores Krieger, a registered nurse and a professor at New York University, and Dora Kunz, a natural healer and a fifth-generation clairvoyant who was president of the Theosophical Society of America from 1975 to 1987.

Dolores Krieger has an interesting cultural background. Krieger's biological father was an Apache and her mother a Mohawk. Born in 1922, she was adopted by a Jewish family as an infant. For the past several decades, she has been a practicing Buddhist. As a Buddhist and a nurse, she regards compassion and healing as fundamental components of her life. She considers the development, practice, and teaching of Therapeutic Touch her life's work.

Krieger was inspired to develop the Therapeutic Touch modality after Dora Kunz, her friend and mentor, brought to her attention the work of Oskar Estebany, a healer who helped improve the medical conditions of both animals and human beings through the use of his hands. Estebany was even able to improve the growth and recovery of plants that had been subjected to poor conditions and harmful substances. To prove that Estebany's laying on of hands was really working, researchers performed blood tests on the animal and human healees before and after Estebany's treatments. The blood test data on mice and humans revealed significant increases in the oxygen carried by red blood cells, a critical factor in healing. Although skeptics claim that Therapeutic Touch works only because of a placebo effect—that is, because the individuals being treated want to believe in its effectiveness—obviously no placebo effect is possible for mice or plants.

Krieger's focus is on each individual's energy field, which she believes can be brought from a state of disarray into a state of balance through the process of Therapeutic Touch. Krieger is currently a professor and researcher at the nursing school of New York University, where Therapeutic Touch is taught as part of the graduate program curriculum. Krieger has trained more than thirty thousand individuals in the practice of Therapeutic Touch since its development in the early 1970s.

Krieger believes that the practice of Therapeutic Touch need not be restricted to health professionals but can be practiced by any individual who is willing to learn the method and apply it appropriately to friends and family members. The practice of Therapeutic Touch is not difficult to learn, with the basics taking about six hours to master. She believes that the power of Therapeutic Touch resides not only in its specialized use as a healing modality but also in its becoming assimilated into our everyday life experience.

WHAT HAPPENS DURING A SESSION OF THERAPEUTIC TOUCH?

When you participate as a receiver, or healee, in a Therapeutic Touch session, you remain fully clothed, removing only your shoes. You are usually seated, and no oil is used. Some healers never make direct contact with your skin, but rather bring their hands close to your body within range of your energy field. In some cases, gentle hands-on contact is also used.

A session lasts up to thirty minutes, although it could be as short as fifteen to twenty minutes. The length of the session depends on the condition of the healee and the amount of work needed to balance and replenish the energy field.

The goal of treatment is for the Therapeutic Touch healer to restore your health and feelings of well-being by sensing and adjusting the energy fields around you. The healer's hands are used to focus and direct the energy, usually in rhythmic and sweeping motions.

A session of Therapeutic Touch involves four processes: centering, assessment, unruffling, and transfer of energy.

Centering

The healer must be centered in order to provide Therapeutic Touch. While waiting for the healer to become centered, you, as the healee, can use this opportunity to center yourself. As the healee, you might be seated or lying down during the centering phase of Therapeutic Touch.

Centering helps both healer and healee prepare for the Therapeutic Touch experience by reducing disturbances in both individuals' energy fields. Disturbances can take the form of negative thoughts and feelings. Negative thoughts and emotions are not confined within the person. Rather, they are exuded through the skin and into our energy fields, affecting everyone around us.

Centering is a personal, calming process that involves ridding oneself of anxiety, tension, and negative thoughts through meditation and concentration. This process can help you quiet your mind, calm your emotions, and relax your body. It may be accomplished through a variety of techniques, for example, by breathing slowly and evenly, by focusing on a sound, or by visualizing a peaceful image or a safe place. There is no one correct way to center yourself. How you become centered is a matter of personal preference. As you practice centering, you will become familiar with techniques that work for you.

It is through centering that the healer is freed from extraneous, irrelevant stimuli and becomes focused on and in tune with the healee's energy field, the focus of treatment. The centering of the healee makes his or her energy field more receptive to Therapeutic Touch. Thus, centering facilitates and deepens the connection between healer and healee.

Assessment

In order to determine the condition and needs of the healee's energy field, the healer examines it quickly and efficiently during the assessment phase of the Therapeutic Touch process. Assessment of the condition of the energy field is accomplished by the passing of the healer's hands over the body of the healee from head to toe, about 2 to 6 inches above the surface of the skin.

The reason for this range of distance is that if the healer's hands touch the healee's body, the assessment could be tainted by distracting influences, including the feel of the healee's clothing or the heat of the skin. Holding the hands too far away will bring them out of range of the healee's energy field. The healer's hands pass over both the front and back of the healee's body. The healee is usually seated, rather than lying down, during the assessment phase of the process. The seated position allows the healer to pass the hands over both the front and back of the healee's body (see Figures 23.1 and 23.2).

Even if your presenting complaint is specific to one part of your body, the energy field of your entire body will be assessed, because a problem in any one area is probably connected to your energy system as a whole.

Imbalances are expressed by the healee's energy field and processed by the healer in a number of forms, including variations in temperature, pulsations, static, other sounds, and even in colors. The entire assessment process

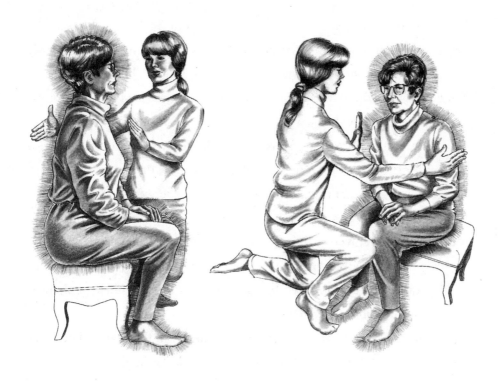

Figure 23.1 and Figure 23.2   Assessing the Energy Field in Therapeutic Touch

lasts only fifteen to thirty seconds. In this modality, swiftly passing over the energy field results in a more accurate assessment than slow movements.

Unruffling

After the assessment is completed, the healer clears the healee's energy field of any static or congestion. This quick, downward sweeping motion, from head to toe, unruffles the healee's energy field, making it receptive for the process of energy transfer, the heart of the Therapeutic Touch process.

Transfer of Energy

The healer's hands are used for the transfer of energy and for stimulating and enhancing the healee's own natural healing ability. Thus, in addition to being provided with new energy, the healee is also provided with the means to continue to renew the energy.

During the transfer of energy, the healer draws on universal energy, which flows from the healer to the healee. The reason the healer draws from universal energy is that using one's own personal energy would quickly lead to depletion of energy and exhaustion in the healer. Knowing that the healer is drawing from universal energy during the energy transfer can help reassure you, as the healee, that you are not taking something from the healer that is vital to that person's well-being. Rather, the energy transfer enhances and rejuvenates both healer and healee.

The healer places the hands several inches from the healee's body and moves them in a manner that directs and modulates the flow of energy to those areas found deficient or blocked during the assessment. The process lasts the number of minutes it takes for the healer to sense that your energy is unblocked, balanced, and flowing freely.

WIDELY ACCEPTED BUT STILL CONTROVERSIAL

This alternative health practice has gained considerable interest, respect, and research funding in a short time. Therapeutic Touch is practiced by more than thirty thousand health care professionals worldwide. More than a hundred thousand people have been trained in Therapeutic Touch techniques. It is practiced in more than thirty countries and is taught at more than eighty universities and hospitals. There are fully accredited master's degree programs that teach the theory and practice of Therapeutic Touch. Numerous doctoral dissertations on the Therapeutic Touch modality have been accepted by accredited universities.

In 1987, Dolores Krieger was awarded the National League of Nursing's prestigious Martha E. Rogers Award for her work on Therapeutic Touch. Therapeutic Touch has been incorporated into the College of Nurses of Ontario 1990 Implementation Standards of Practice. In early 1994, the U.S. National Institute of Health awarded a research grant to study Therapeutic Touch. Even more recently, the Department of Defense, through the Uniformed Services University of the Health Sciences, awarded researchers at the University of Alabama Burn Center more than $350,000 to study the effectiveness of Therapeutic Touch on patients with burns.

The reason for the widespread acceptance of the healing power of Therapeutic Touch is that its recipients report that it works. In addition to claims made by thousands of individuals that they feel better after the procedure, there is clinical and scientific evidence of its effectiveness. Health practitioners have observed clinically that acute conditions and wounds heal faster with the application of Therapeutic Touch.

Scientific evidence of the positive impact of Therapeutic Touch on the injuries and infections of young children and animals demonstrates that the healing power of this process is not due to just a placebo effect or the human adult recipient's belief that the process will be helpful. Physical healing is promoted by hemoglobin in the blood. In her milestone study published in 1975, Krieger demonstrated a significantly greater increase in the average hemoglobin level of a group of patients who received Therapeutic Touch than in that of a control group of patients who received routine nursing care with no Therapeutic Touch.

Benefits of Therapeutic Touch

Increased relaxation.

Pain reduction.

Faster healing from acute conditions, illness, and injury.

Faster healing and relief from infections and congestion.

Lessening of hypertension, headaches, and other stress-induced psychosomatic conditions.

Increased relaxation and serenity for individuals with serious chronic conditions.

Quicker healing and pain reduction for postsurgical and burn patients who cannot tolerate direct contact with their skin.

In spite of the widespread acceptance of the effectiveness of Therapeutic Touch, there is controversy surrounding this modality. Because you cannot see an energy field and cannot prove that you feel one, many skeptics claim that human energy fields and universal energy do not exist. In April 1998, a study was conducted by a nine-year-old girl that bolstered the skeptics' views. Emily Rosa made history by being the youngest person to have research published in the *Journal of the American Medical Association*. For a school project, Rosa designed an experiment to test the validity of Therapeutic Touch. In her study, she asked twenty-one Therapeutic Touch practitioners to put their hands through a cardboard screen and, with their sight blocked, asked them to identify which of their hands were near one of hers. More than half the healers failed to make a correct identification (*The Times*, April 2, 1998).

In the same newspaper article, it was reported that a family practitioner, Robert P. Blankfield, M.D., received in 1997 a grant in the amount of $7,500 from the Ohio Academy of Family Physicians to conduct a study on the effectiveness of Therapeutic Touch on one hundred subjects who suffered from carpal tunnel syndrome, an increasingly common, painful disorder. A nurse who had practiced Therapeutic Touch for more than ten years in hospitals, nursing homes, and wellness centers with successful results was quoted as saying that if this alternative treatment did not produce positive results, it would have died by now.

UNIQUE BENEFITS

Therapeutic Touch promotes relaxation, reduces pain, and can accelerate the healing process for both physical injuries and acute illnesses, including infections and congestion. It has also been shown to be effective in reducing hypertension, headaches, and other stress-induced psychosomatic disorders.

Although Therapeutic Touch has not been shown to change the course of chronic conditions like cancer, the use of this modality has helped victims of cancer and other life-threatening illnesses feel more relaxed and serene during the difficult treatments and emotional turmoil that accompany such diseases.

Because it is not necessary to touch the body physically, a unique benefit of this method is that it can be applied in situations in which the receiver may not be able to tolerate contact—for example, postsurgical patients and burn victims. Such patients have reported experiencing soothing relief, and their injuries have healed more quickly with the addition of Therapeutic Touch to their treatment plans.

Conclusion

You have reached the end of your journey through our book on bodywork and massage. We hope that you now feel equipped to begin or to continue your exploration of the modalities that suit your needs.

As we have reiterated throughout the book, bodywork and massage are not a substitute for medical treatments. However, physical and mental health as well as personal and spiritual growth can be enhanced through the power of touch. Your willingness to provide an accurate history and description of your needs will make the process safe and satisfying.

The practitioner or giver you choose is perhaps as important as the types of bodywork and massage you decide to pursue. Touch is personal. It is important not only that the practitioner be qualified but also that you feel a rapport. The relationship between giver and receiver is a factor in the outcome of treatment. Whether the giver provides relaxation, pain relief, or universal energy, your comfort level and trust in the giver will play a critical role in the healing process.

Appendix A provides key information about the modalities in summary form. You will see at a glance the overlap and the differences on various dimensions. Appendix B and the bibliography that follow are intended to give you the opportunity to find out even more than we could include in the limited space of one book. Enjoy your continuing journey in the fascinating world of bodywork and massage.

Key Features of the Modalities at a Glance

The information provided in this appendix has been organized into a simple format so that you can determine at a glance the key features of the bodywork and massage modalities. You can use the summary chart provided for different purposes. For example, you could examine every feature for a particular modality, or you could compare one or more modalities according to some or all of the features included. You will notice that there are areas of overlap as well as differences among the modalities.

TRANSLATION OF THE ABBREVIATIONS

Some of the items in the chart that follows are abbreviated. To help you read the items correctly and without guesswork, all abbreviations are explained:

Clothing   Clothing worn while receiving the modality:

    U   Undressed or underwear only

    L   Light, comfortable clothing

    C   Clothed

Lub   Whether or not massage oil or any other type of lubrication is used in this modality:

    vl   Only very light use of lubrication at times

Duration   The number of minutes per session is indicated. Where there is a range, e.g., 30 to 60, the length of the session depends on the needs, health status, or wishes of the client.

	TOUCH	CLOTHING	LUB	SERIES	DURATION
Swedish massage	Soothing	U or L	Yes	No	30 to 90
Infant massage	Light	U	Yes	No	Varies
Sports massage	Deep	U or L	Yes	No	Varies
Geriatric massage	Light	U or L or C	Yes	No	30
Myofascial release	Deep	U or L	No	No	30 to 90
Neuromuscular therapy	Deep	U or L	No	No	15 to 60
Shiatsu	Deep	L	No	No	30 to 90
Reflexology	Deep	C	No/vl	No	20 to 60
Trager Approach	Light	L	No/vl	No	30 to 60
Manual lymph drainage	Light	U or L	Yes	No	30 to 60
Craniosacral therapy	Light	C	No	No	45 to 60
Rosen Method	Light	U or L	No	No	60
Rolfing	Deep	U	No	Yes	60 to 90
Hellerwork	Deep	U	No	Yes	90
Alexander Technique	Light	C	No	No	30 to 60
Feldenkrais Method	Light	C	No	No	45 to 60
Reiki	None/Light	C	No	No	30 to 90
Polarity Therapy	Light	L	No	No	30 to 90
Therapeutic Touch	None	C	No	No	15 to 30

Resources

The purpose of this appendix is to provide you with a list of resources for obtaining more information about the different approaches, training, and how to locate a practitioner in your geographic area.

THE ALEXANDER TECHNIQUE

North American Society of Teachers of the Alexander Technique (NASTAT)
P.O. Box 112484
Tacoma, WA 98411-2484
(206) 627-3766 or 1-800-473-0620

The American Center for the Alexander Technique, Inc.
129 West 67th Street
New York, NY 10023
(212) 799-0468

CRANIOSACRAL THERAPY

The Upledger Institute
11211 Prosperity Farms Road
Palm Beach, FL 33410
1-800-233-5880

THE FELDENKRAIS METHOD

The Feldenkrais Foundation
P.O. Box 70157
Washington, DC 20088
(301) 656-1548

The Feldenkrais Guild
706 SW Ellsworth St.
P.O. Box 489
Albany, OR 97321-0143
(503) 926-0981 or 1-800-775-2118
Fax: (503) 926-0572

Feldenkrais Resources
830 Bancroft Way
Berkeley, CA 94710
(510) 540-7600 or 1-800-765-1907

GERIATRIC MASSAGE

Deitrich Miesler
P.O. Box 1629
Guerneville, CA 95446

Day-Break Geriatric Massage Project
P.O. Box 1815
Sebastopol, CA 95473

HELLERWORK

Hellerwork, Inc.
406 Berry Street
Mount Shasta, CA 96067
(916) 926-2500 or 1-800-392-3900

INFANT MASSAGE

Association of Infant Massage
Instructors
P.O. Box 16103
Portland, OR 97216-0103

Gentle Touch
4302 20th Avenue
Moline, IL 61265

MANUAL LYMPH DRAINAGE (MLD)

Dr. Vodder School–North America
P.O. Box 5701
Victoria, BC
Canada V8R 6S8
Tel. and Fax: (250) 598-9862

North American Vodder Association
of Lymphatic Therapy (NAVALT)
(888) 462-8258

MYOFASCIAL RELEASE THERAPY

MFR Treatment Center & Seminars
Routes 30 and 252
10 South Leopard Road, Suite 1
Paoli, PA 19301
(610) 644-0136 or 1-800-327-2425

POLARITY THERAPY

American Polarity Therapy
Association
2888 Bluff Street
Suite 149
Boulder, CO 80301
(303) 545-2080
Fax: (303) 545-2161

REFLEXOLOGY

International Institute of Reflexology
P.O. Box 12642
St. Petersburg, FL 33733-2642
(813) 343-4811
Fax: (813) 381-2807

American Reflexology Certification
Board
P.O. Box 620607
Littleton, CO 80162
(303) 933-6921

REIKI

The Reiki Alliance
P.O. Box 41
Cataldo, ID 83810-1041
(208) 682-3535
Fax: (208) 682-4848

The Center for Reiki Training
29209 Northwestern Highway, No. 592
Southfield, MI 48034
1-800-332-8112
Fax: (810) 948-9534

ROLFING

The Rolf Institute
205 Canyon Boulevard
P.O. Box 1868
Boulder, CO 80302-1868
(303) 449-5903 or 1-800-530-8875
Fax: (303) 449-5978
E-mail: Rolfinst@aol.com

THE ROSEN METHOD

Eastern United States and Canada
Rosen Center East
P.O. Box 5004
Westport, CT 06881-5004
(203) 319-1090 or 1-800-484-9832
Fax: (203) 319-0032

Rocky Mountain area and Southwest
Rosen Method Center Southwest
P.O. Box 344
Santa Fe, NM 87504
(505) 982-7149

West Coast
Rosen Method–The Berkeley Center
825 Bancroft Avenue, Suite A
Berkeley, CA 94710
(510) 845-6606

Canada
Rosen Method–Cascadia Centre
(604) 885-0487

All other areas
**Rosen Method Professional
Association (RMPA)**
2550 Shattuck Avenue
Box 49
Berkeley, CA 94704
(510) 644-4166

SHIATSU

Acupressure Institute
1533 Shattuck Avenue
Berkeley, CA 94709
(510) 845-1059 or 1-800-442-2232

American Shiatsu Association
295 Huntington Avenue
Boston, MA 02015
(617) 236-2286

Ohashi Institute
Kinderhook, NY 12106
(518) 758-6879
Fax: (518) 758-6809

SWEDISH, SPORTS, GERIATRIC, AND NEUROMUSCULAR THERAPY

Alliance of Massage Therapists, Inc.
c/o Swedish Institute
226 West 26th Street
New York, NY 10001
(212) 736-1100

American Massage Therapy Association (AMTA)
820 Davis Street, Suite 100
Evanston, IL 60201-4444
(708) 864-0123
Fax: (708) 864-1178

THERAPEUTIC TOUCH

Nurse Healers—Professional Associates, Inc.
P.O. Box 44
Allison Park, PA 15101-0444
(412) 355-8476

Pumpkin Hollow Foundation
RR 1, Box 135
Craryville, NY 12521
(518) 325-3583 or (518) 325-7105

The Therapeutic Touch Network
P.O. Box 85551
875 Eglinton Avenue West
Toronto, Ontario
Canada M6C 4A8
(416) 65-TOUCH

THE TRAGER APPROACH

The Trager Institute
33 Millwood Street
Mill Valley, CA 94941-2091
(415) 388-2688
Fax: (415) 388-2710
E-mail: Trageradmin@trager.com

Bibliography

There are many valuable books and articles on various aspects and modalities of bodywork and massage. We have chosen a representative sample to include in this bibliography.

Baginski, Bodo J., and Shalila Sharamon. *Reiki—Universal Life Energy.* Mendocino, Calif.: Life Rhythm, 1988.

Barnes, John F., P.T. "The Myofascial Release Approach: The Missing Link." *Massage* 49 (May/June 1994): 36–38, 40–45.

———."The Myofascial Release Approach, Part II: The Mind-Body Connection." *Massage* 50 (July/Aug. 1994): 58, 60–64.

Beck, Mark. *The Theory and Practice of Therapeutic Massage.* Bronx, N.Y.: Milady Publishing Company, 1988.

Bond, Mary. *Rolfing Movement Integration: A Self-Help Approach to Balancing the Body.* Rochester, Vt.: Healing Arts Press, 1993.

Calvert, Robert. "Dolores Krieger, Ph.D., and Her Therapeutic Touch." *Massage* 47 (Jan./Feb. 1994): 56–60.

———."The Feldenkrais Method—The Man, His Work and the Training." *Massage* 47 (Jan./Feb. 1994): 30–36.

Chopra, Deepak, M.D. *Boundless Energy.* New York: Harmony Books, 1995.

Claire, Thomas. *Bodywork.* New York: Morrow, 1995.

Conningham, Bill. "The Alexander Technique: Learn to Use Your Body with Ease." *Massage* 63 (Sept./Oct. 1996): 20–25.

Cottingham, John T. *Healing Through Touch: A History and a Review of the Physiological Evidence.* Boulder, Colo.: Rolf Institute, 1985.

Dienstfrey, Harris. *Where the Mind Meets the Body.* New York HarperCollins, 1991.

Dychtwald, Ken. *Bodymind.* Los Angeles: Jeremy Tarcher, 1986.

Feitis, Rosemary (ed.). *Ida Rolf Talks about Rolfing and Physical Reality.* Boulder, Colo.: Rolf Institute, 1978.

Feldenkrais, Moshe. *Awareness Through Movement: Easy-to-do Health Exercises to Improve Your Posture, Vision, Imagination and Personal Awareness.* San Francisco: Harper & Row, 1992.

———.*The Potent Self: A Guide to Spontaneity.* San Francisco: HarperCollins, 1985.

Felton, John (ed.). *Hands-on Healing.* Emmaus, Penn.: Rodale Press, 1989.

Field, Tiffany, S. Schanberg, F. Scafidi, et. al. "Tactile/Kinesthetic Stimulation Effects on Preterm Neonates." *Pediatrics* 77 (May 1986): 654–658.

Gray, John. *Your Guide to the Alexander Technique.* New York: St. Martin's Press, 1990.

Juhan, Deane, M.A. *An Introduction to Trager Psychophysical Integration and Mentastics Movement Education.* Mill Valley, Calif.: Trager Institute, 1989.

King, Robert, K. *Performance Massage.* Windsor, Ontario, Canada: Human Kinetics Publishers, 1993.

Knaster, Mirka. "The View from John E. Upledger's Cranium." *Massage Therapy Journal* 37 no. 2 (Summer 1998): 57–60, 62.

Krieger, Dolores. *Accepting Your Power to Heal: The Personal Practice of Therapeutic Touch.* Santa Fe, N. Mex.: Bear & Co., Inc., 1993.

Krieger, Dolores. *Living the Therapeutic Touch: Healing as a Lifestyle.* New York: Dodd, Mead, 1987.

———.*The Therapeutic Touch: How to Use Your Hands to Help or to Heal.* New York: Prentice Hall, 1979.

Laskin, Jack. "Milton Trager, M.D.: The Master at 86." *Massage* 51 (Sept./Oct. 1994): 26, 28–29.

Leboyer, Frederick. *Loving Hands.* New York: Alfred A. Knopf, 1979.

Macrae, Janet. *Therapeutic Touch: A Practical Guide.* New York: Knopf, 1988.

Maisal, Edward (ed.). *The Alexander Technique: The Essential Writings of F. Matthias Alexander.* New York: Lyle Stuart, 1990.

Masunaga, Shizuto, with Wataru Ohashi. *Zen Shiatsu.* Tokyo and New York: Japan Publications, Inc., 1977.

McClure, Vimala Schneider. *Infant Massage—A Handbook for Loving Parents* (Revised). New York: Bantam, 1989.

Meagher, John, with Pat Boughton. *Sportsmassage: A Complete Program for Increasing Performance and Endurance in Fifteen Popular Sports.* Barringtown, N.Y.: Station Hill Press, 1990.

Montagu, Ashley. *Touching: The Human Significance of the Skin,* Third Edition. New York: Harper & Row, 1986.

Nelson, Dawn. *Compassionate Touch.* Barrytown, N.Y.: Station Hill Press, 1994.

Rice, Ruth. "Premature Infants Respond to Sensory Stimulation." *American Psychiatric Association Monitor* 6 (Nov. 1975): 8.

Rosen, Marion, with Sue Brenner. *The Rosen Method of Movement.* Berkeley, Calif.: North Atlantic Books, 1991.

Schwartz, Don, Ph.D. "What Could Be Lighter? The Work of Milton Trager, M.D." *Massage* 67 (May/June 1997): 56–58, 60, 63.

Segal, Maybelle. *Reflexology.* Hollywood, Calif.: Melvin Powers Wilshire Book Company, 1976.

Serepca, Beth Anne. "Interview with Tiffany Field, Ph.D." *Massage* 63 (Sept./Oct. 1996): 44–48.

Siegel, Alan. *Polarity Therapy.* San Leandro, Calif.: Prism Press, 1987.

Stolzoft, Russell. "The Rolfing Method: The Evolution of Structural Integration." *Massage* 70 (Nov./Dec. 1997): 34–38.

Stone, Randolph. *Polarity Therapy: The Complete Collected Works on This Revolutionary Healing Art by the Originator of the System.* Sebastopol, Calif.: CRCS Publications, 1986.

Tappan, Frances M. *Healing Massage Techniques,* Second Edition. Norwalk, Conn.: Appleton & Lange, 1988.

Trager, Milton, M.D., with Cathy Guadagno, Ph.D. *Trager Mentastics: Movement as a Way to Agelessness.* Barrytown, N.Y.: Station Hill Press, 1987.

Upledger, John E., D.O., O.M.M. "Initial Observations of the Craniosacral System." *Massage* 65 (Jan./Feb. 1997): 91, 93, 96, 99.

———."Tissue Memory, Energy Cysts and Healing Energy." *Massage* 67 (May/June 1997): 91–93, 95–98.

Walker, Peter. *The Book of Baby Massage.* New York: Simon & Schuster, 1988.

Index